1998

the
world's
best-kept
diet secrets

THE
WORLD'S
BEST-KEPT
DIET SECRETS

Lose Weight Quickly, Safely and Permanently

DIANE IRONS

Sourcebooks, Inc.
Naperville, IL

Published by: Sourcebooks
P.O. Box 372, Naperville, Illinois 60566
(630) 961-3900
FAX: (630) 961-2168

Irons, Diane 1949-
     The world's best-kept diet secrets : lose weight quickly, safely,
  and permanently / Diane Irons
        p. cm.
     Includes index.
     ISBN 1-57071-375-8 (alk. paper)
     1. Weight loss. I. Title.
RM222.2.I76 1998
613.2'5—dc21   98-21342
                                                                                              CIP

Printed and bound in the United States of America.

10   9   8   7   6   5   4   3   2   1

Table of Contents

Acknowledgments viii

Introduction ix

Chapter 1: Getting Started 1

Chapter 2: Dieting Myths 21

Chapter 3: Tricks and Tools 39

Chapter 4: Food Choices 57

Chapter 5: Looking Good While Going Down 67

Chapter 6: Secrets of Models and Celebrities 81

Chapter 7: Diet Emergencies 97

Chapter 8: Supplements 109

Chapter 9: Exercise 127

Chapter 10: Special Problems 143

Chapter 11: Intimacy and Weight 165

Chapter 12: Children and Weight 173

Chapter 13: Holidays, Vacations, and Other Trip-Ups . 179

Chapter 14: Success Stories 195

Chapter 15: Bargains and Freebies 213

Chapter 16: Other Weight Loss Options 227

Chapter 17: Shortcuts 235

Chapter 18: Questions 245

Chapter 19: Recipes under 200 Calories 257

A Final Word 309

About the Author 310

Index 311

Dedication

To David and Kirk

Acknowledgments

So many people have contributed to this book by sharing their stories, their expertise, their time, and most importantly, their hearts. My deepest appreciation goes to my many colleagues and friends, who upon hearing of my quest for concrete answers to the conundrum of dieting and weight loss, led me to the most powerful and precise resources.

I am extremely grateful to my publicist and dear friend, Renee Calomino, for her dedication and intuitive knowledge of my intentions. I consider our relationship an invaluable gift in both my life and my work.

My deep thanks to my publisher, Dominique Raccah, for trusting in my message of hope, reason, and logic in the absurd world of image.

My indebtedness to my editor, Todd Stocke, for refining my body of work and assuring its accuracy and practicality.

Finally, there are not enough words in which to thank my husband, David, my life's love, and my son, Kirk, my "lucky star."

Introduction

When it comes to losing weight and keeping it off, what really works? I have been looking for the answer ever since I started modeling at the age of thirteen and had to fight my own weight problems. I looked to the most beautiful bodies in the business to give me the answers and direction. When I became a reporter and image consultant, regardless of the story I was covering, at the end of the interview, if there was a body I admired, I wanted to know how it happened. Have you always been slim? If not, how did you get the weight off? How do you stay so disciplined? What do you eat? What do you avoid? Is your family slim? How do you lose weight quickly when a film or modeling job comes up? What's your favorite low calorie recipe? Usually, when the microphone comes down, the reserves fall away and the stars shared their secrets with me.

It was not just celebrities who intrigued me. My nationally broadcast "lifestyle" shows featured "real" people who shared with me both their triumphs and tragedies. Again, their weight played important roles in their relationships, self-esteem, and career choices. In my research for this book, I interviewed men and women who spent countless dollars on books, pills, pricey diet and exercise programs, and other promises. I tracked down friends who had friends with important life changing stories.

This book is a compilation of tips from famous celebrities and "real" people. I have talked to trainers to find out the best exercises and equipment for the least money. I have worked with nutritionists, physicians, and chemists to find the natural supplements that are important aids to weight loss.

I hope I have covered everything. Probably like you, I have tired of diet books that tell one story, one struggle, one philosophy. Although these books are well-intentioned, what worked for me, him, or her may not drive you to your own answer. My hope is that you will draw on your own inspiration and create your own lifestyle changes from my pursuits.

In order to get the intimate stories in this book, I had to promise my subjects total anonymity, so I have identified them only by their first name, age, and the amount of weight they have lost. Weight losses ranged from just 10 pounds to almost 200 pounds, but the weight must have stayed off at least five years to be included. Like many of us, my contacts had often lost and regained weight several times before finally reaching their permanent goals.

Use this book to find the keys to success that exist within the framework of your own personality. These are the tools and information you will need to get there, but it is you who will do the work and reap the fabulous rewards to come.

Chapter One

Getting Started

So What's the Secret?

Diets Are Like Spokes on a Wheel

When we hear about someone who's lost weight and kept it off, we all want to know how they did it. What was the secret to their success? I have spent years attempting to unlock these secrets in my work as an image researcher and journalist. From my "other" life in modeling, I have been witness to great successes of permanent weight loss as well as seeing highly lucrative careers ruined by food obsessions.

Let me set you straight before we get started. I did not find one diet that is going to work for everyone. I have interviewed hundreds of individuals who have successfully lost weight and kept it off. They did it by charting their own course. Most diet books are one person's experience or opinion, and at the very least anecdotal. This storytelling of "what worked for me" has sold a lot of books. Physicians also put forth dieting advice which is theory-based, and did not work for the majority of the successful dieters I interviewed. These diets failed because they were too complicated to follow, too prohibitive, or too expensive. Sometimes they worked for the short term, but could not sustain long-term results. These doctors are not gods or gurus, and my interviews conclude that diets are more about lifestyle change than simply a matter of science and chemistry. Diets are about life.

What's Your Story?

It comes as no surprise that each dieter has a different philosophy of "ideal" weight. Rather than following weight charts, successful dieters chose to rely on criteria such as the weight at which they felt their most comfortable, pre-pregnancy weights, etc. Their stories included cruelty, abandonment, embarrassment, and discrimination.

Playing Mind Games

When I asked people their initial feelings before embarking on a diet program, the overwhelming response was "anxiety," a reply echoed by both successful and failed dieters. Dieters feel enormous trepidation and a fear of being overwhelmed. It hits them hardest when they start out, no matter what their size, goal, or planned regime.

"I was afraid that my obsession with chocolate would not allow me to get to my final goal. It was only recognizing that I could have one piece of chocolate a day that let me get through it."

Mary, age 38, 25 pounds lost

"My fears were due to my extreme hate of exercise. I knew that exercise was necessary for weight loss, but for me it was just too overwhelming to think about getting geared up for a diet and exercise program at the same time. My solution was to not join a gym, but start walking whenever I could. I got hooked on it, and now I run three miles a day and love how it makes me feel."

Frank, age 45, 53 pounds lost

2

Take Charge

You need to come to the decision that food has dictated how you live your life for far too long. It probably has colored every component of your daily activity. Those who have found their weight loss to be successful permanently talk about a feeling of power, where previously there was only powerlessness.

Wipe the Slate Clean

Successful weight loss begins with the end of doubts, regrets, and remorse—no more of "what if?" "why did I?" and "if only." It really doesn't matter what you did yesterday or ten years ago. It doesn't matter how old you are or how many pounds you want to lose. To accomplish your goal, it is important for you to set your site on mini goals. Losing eighty pounds is tremendously scary, and yet making yourself ten pounds lighter is not only attainable, but a goal you can live with for now.

Pace Yourself

Eat what you want, and eat it when you want. The reason why diet programs have such a high failure rate is partly due to their regimentation. Taking away your favorite foods only makes you feel even more deprived. You won't go too long before those cravings for pizza and chocolate overcome your every waking minute. Look, even if you hate brussel sprouts, any diet that said you could never have them again would make you think about them all the time. Next thing you know, you'll be craving them. You'll be hitting the grocery stores looking for brussel sprouts!

There is no "bad" food, and although some foods are better than others, there are no "good" foods.

Get those words out of your vocabulary, and keep them out. Everyone has their own rhythm that feels right to them. Also, only you know when you're truly hungry. Eating by the clock is just not workable for most successful dieters.

Start a Food Diary

The only way you'll win this battle is to figure out what triggers your overeating. Even if you head into a binge, putting your feelings down on paper will create a commonality that will help you understand the nature of your weight problems. Calories have a way of creeping up. Research done by the American Dietetic Association found that dieters who were not successful after countless weight loss efforts were underestimating their calories by as much as 300 percent. They also thought they exercised much more than they really did. If it's too hard to keep a daily journal, at least try to keep

track of two weekdays and one weekend day. Note such things as mood, fat and calorie content of what you eat, what you were doing or feeling before you ate, and how you felt afterwards (satisfied, sad, mad, etc.).

Know Your Body Fat

Your weight is important, but the amount of fat in your body is equally important. Combining both gives a more accurate picture of overall body fitness. If you have an acceptable weight but too much body fat, your health could be in jeopardy. The USDA recommendation is that no more than 30 percent of your daily caloric intake come from fat.

Here's how to measure:
1. Using a millimeter ruler, pinch the fold of skin directly in front of your armpit, vertically in at the front of your thigh, and vertically an inch to the

side of your belly button. Hold the ruler away from your body, as straight as possible.

2. Add all three measurements together.

3. Your total should be no higher than 100. Higher than that means that you have more than 30 percent body fat.

Do You Know Your BMI?

The body mass index (BMI) measures the relationship between your weight and your height. Here's how you find yours:

1. Multiply your weight in pounds by .45 to get kilos.

2. Take your height in inches and multiply by 0.0254 to get meters.

3. Multiply that number by itself.

4. Divide this into your weight in kilos. This is your BMI. The accepted healthy range is from 19 to 25 according to the National Examination Survey.

How Much Should You Weigh?

Forget the complicated chart! An easy way to figure out what you should weigh is to allow 100 pounds for the first five feet of height and five pounds for each additional inch. Most charts calculate that ten pounds below that is just about right for small frames, and ten pounds above is normal for larger frames. But don't get married to that. You know where you feel your healthiest.

There are lots of other criteria to consider also. Yours might be getting back into your wedding or prom dress. With most people I've interviewed, they usually cite their high school weight as their ideal. From what I've observed, it's been self-sabotaging to get stuck at a certain weight. However, adhering to a weight range seems to work for most successful dieters no matter how much they've lost. For some it's ten pounds and for others it's just five. I remember interviewing the late Ava Gabor who weighed herself twice a day. If she weighed more than one pound than the previous day's weight she cut out all bread and dessert that day. She told me that she just couldn't trust herself otherwise. That's pretty stringent, but is pretty typical of anyone I've ever interviewed whose career was based on their looks.

Don't Get Too Technical

The problem with most diet books and diet programs is that they are so complicated and difficult to follow that the dieters I interviewed found themselves constantly having to think about what they ate. This result proved a negative for the majority of them. They were literally consumed with thoughts of food, which caused them to overeat.

"I've been on more 'stylized' diets than I want to count. Trying to figure out what to eat next made me crazy! I had food on the mind all the time. Only when I could finally sit down to a meal and eat what appealed to me at that very moment did I feel like a 'real' person."

Tasha, age 48, 60 pounds lost

Tasha is typical of successful dieters who told me that choosing foods that felt "right" at the time, were convenient, etc., were what they needed. Some even labeled it "self-permission." These dieters were more successful when they discovered the tools they needed for their weight loss. They regarded the more complex diet programs as complicated architectural blueprints that made no sense to their lives or lifestyles.

Listen to Your Body

Your body will signal you with what is wrong and what it needs. Sometimes it will scream at you for help. For example, women report craving certain foods (usually chocolate) about a week before their menstrual cycles. Research indicates that this is due to a deficiency of magnesium. In another person, fatigue may mean that more protein is needed in their diet. Also, craving "comfort" foods like bread, pastry, or crackers could simply indicate boredom or stress.

"I can't tell you the number of days I would come home from a particularly bad day at work, and head directly to that bag of chips or crackers. More times than I care to admit, it would be before taking my coat off or greeting my family. Learning

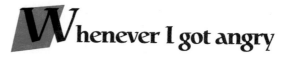

Whenever I got angry

I would eat and eat until the feelings went away. My head would tell me not to do it. On an intellectual level, I knew what was happening, but I was powerless to the quick fix.

Peter, age 64, 110 pounds lost

to meditate for ten minutes after work helped me to avoid an entire night of binging."

Sid, age 39, 82 pounds lost

"Realizing that taking two aspirin alleviated my headaches more efficiently (and with a lot less calories) than a pint of ice cream or an entire cheesecake allowed me to take charge of my health and my weight."

Marsha, age 52, 36 pounds lost

Develop a Reward System

Successful dieters have found that having something to look forward to at the end of each milestone (first five pounds, getting through a tough weekend, etc.) helped to mentally and emotionally shorten the cycles of long-term success.

"I realized that I had to look at myself in an entirely different way. Somehow over the years I had put myself on the shelf and didn't feel I was worthy enough, partly because of my weight, to treat myself to the 'little luxuries.' So even though I had a tremendous amount of weight to lose, I began to act like those high maintenance babes I had so long been envious of. For every five pounds I lost, I had my nails done (even pedicures), had my hair highlighted, and made inexpensive 'bauble' purchases. They made me feel good about myself, which were feelings that I had long ago forgotten. Looking forward to those little rewards helped me to stay on track during the toughest days."

Marge, age 44, 77 pounds lost

Accept the Consequences

Just as important as rewarding themselves through the milestones of their diet, it was equally beneficial for dieters to accept some form of retribution for slipping. For some it was as simple as not allowing themselves their daily treat for two or three days, while for others it was more punitive.

"I had to take 'just this once' completely out of my vocabulary. When I went off my diet I would literally punish myself. I would climb 5 floors to my job, make my own coffee rather than buying it, etc. I had to feel that there was going to be more of a cause and effect than just gaining back the weight. I usually incorporated something that would make up for my 'slip up.' It worked for me."

Alan, age 27, 48 pounds lost

It's a Gift You Give Yourself

Think of your weight loss program as the most important gift you have ever given yourself. Only when you take away the "poor me routine" can you

really just grow up and get on with it. Now is the time to experience new tastes. Enjoy the entire experience of eating, and get the most from every morsel. This will eliminate feelings of deprivation.

Talk Back to Your Head

When something goes wrong in our lives, those voices in our head start in. They try to tell us that the only way we'll get over that disappointment or loneliness is with the antidote of food. Tell yourself that you've had these feelings before, and you've lived through it. No amount of food will take away these feelings. In fact, it will only make you feel worse afterward. Then start talking yourself into a better body.

Gender Differences

"Women tend to binge when they are angry or sad, or they use food as a source of comfort when alone or depressed. Obese men were found to binge in positive social situations when celebrating or encouraged by others to eat."

—*Elle* magazine

Create a Contract

Take the time to write out a contract with yourself. These 10 rules are a good start for terms you can live up to. Add your own resolutions to this list if you'd like. Take it out whenever you are tempted to break the terms of the contract.

1. I resolve to eat only when I am truly hungry.

2. I resolve to try a new fruit or vegetable.

3. I resolve to treat myself to a forbidden food once a week.

4. I resolve to limit consumption of diet soda and other chemicals.

5. I resolve to drink 8 to 10 glasses of water daily.

6. I resolve to exercise at least 3 times a week.

7. I resolve to replace a red meat meal with tofu.

8. I resolve to accept responsibility for my actions.

9. I resolve to think before I eat.

10. I resolve to take it one day at a time.

My name:_____

My current weight:_____

My goal weight:_____

Reason for losing weight:_____

Signed:_____

Date:_____

Understand Why You Overeat

Everyone knows that food is a great tranquilizer. It creates a buffer zone from the hurts and issues that plague everyone's life experiences. Understanding why they turn to food rather than solving the problems has worked for the chronic binge eaters I interviewed.

"My weight gain came when my last child left for college. I was left with an emptiness that I filled with food. The foods that I chose were the typical comfort foods like cakes, cookies, and the creamiest pastries I could find. Fifty pounds later I finally came to terms with it, and replaced the 'empty foods' with my 'empty nest' realization."

Bunny, age 56, 50 pounds lost

"When I married my husband I weighed 115 pounds. At 5'4" I wore a size seven and thought that I had a pretty good body. My husband never complimented me, but continually put me up against other women. This affected my esteem in such a way that I started to eat as a way of getting back at him. The more he criticized, the more I ate. When he finally left me I weighed in at 188 pounds. When I realized that I could never base my appearance on other's expectations, and that I was good 'as is,' I was able to take control of my weight and my life."

Portia, age 36, 62 pounds lost

Stop Fighting Nature

When setting your goal weight, try not to squeeze into some "ideal" mold that you've seen in the movies or a fashion magazine. If you've never been a size four, chances are you are not meant to be that small.

11

Be Aware of Seasonal Challenges

A lot of us gain weight during the colder months. The average gain is between 5 to 7 pounds, usually gained around the holidays. The type of foods we eat also make a major contribution to this weight gain. We are less likely to reach for that salad when we're chilly. The dieters I interviewed told me that their biggest diet challenges came during the winter months. Outside activities are usually curtailed, and exercise programs drop off.

"I couldn't get my body warm enough. I guess I tried to compensate for this by reaching for heavy foods. When I tried to warm myself up with coffee, it just made me jittery, and again, I would use food to calm me down. Now that I've lost the weight, I keep bouillon cubes on hand, and sip broth throughout the day. At just six calories a cup, I keep myself warm and satisfied all day long."

Paul, age 47, 23 pounds lost

"I hate the whole gym scene, but I couldn't get myself out the door in the freezing temperatures and on icy roads to walk the hour I do in nice weather. Investing in a treadmill and keeping it in sight was a lifesaver in keeping my weight off."

Moe, age 33, 18 pounds lost

Check That Stress Level

Almost everyone, no matter what their lifestyle, no matter how much money in the bank, told me that one of the greatest challenges to their weight loss was coping with stress. Whether it was a client's demands, the kids fighting, or even trying to balance the checkbook, a quick trip to the kitchen was the only way they could diffuse the tension building up inside. So we eat, and get even more stressed out.

The weight loss industry makes profits of over $40 billion a year!

Change Your Relationship with Food

Dieters who maintain long-term weight loss have had to come to terms with the role that food plays in their daily lives. Only when they were able to put food back into its proper place were they able to not only lose the excess pounds, but also resume a normal lifestyle.

"The whole issue of food was taking up too much of my time. There were more days than I care to count when I would wake up thinking of food, praying to God to keep me away from the frig. I was unable to work, to think, even to move. Previously, I had been able to quit smoking and overcome a prescription drug dependency. This was harder because obviously I couldn't eliminate food from my life."

Chuck, age 26, 120 pounds lost

Expect a Rocky Road

The final success is the acceptance that there is bound to be failure along the way to reaching your goal. Eliminating that "all or nothing" attitude and planning for those inevitable glitches will allow you to look at the long range plan you've made. When you do break your diet, you're able to pick yourself up, dust yourself off, and get going again.

13

"When I would eat one cookie, I would figure that I had blown the whole day, so instead of eating just that one cookie, I would devour the entire box. Now I allow myself to have one, even two cookies, and not feel that I've taken a big setback. Allowing myself to enjoy the occasional treat keeps me from feeling alienated from society."

Pat, age 34, 40 pounds lost

Never Skip Meals

Skipping any meal sets you up to overeat at the next meal. With that said, though, many dieters did not adhere to three meals a day. Some ate just twice a day while others chose to eat six mini-meals throughout the day. The key is to eat at regular intervals.

"I have a problem of going in and out of the refrigerator and the kitchen cabinets all day long. What worked for me was taking the models from *Sports Illustrated*, cutting off their heads, and sticking my head on top of their bodies. I stuck a picture on each of my 'dangerous' cabinets as well as on the refrigerator."

Sandy, age 30, 25 pounds lost

Don't Call It a Diet

People who have and kept off the weight they lost have done so by pretty much sticking to whatever tools they used to take the weight off in the first place. Even after reaching their goals, successful dieters continued to watch the fat content of the foods they ate, measured portions, and maintained an exercise program.

"As soon as I started going back to my old style of eating, the weight started climbing again. What keeps my weight at bay is using the program I used to lose the weight during the week, and enjoying some extras on the weekend. Yeah, come Monday I may be a couple of pounds up, but I know that it will come off by getting right back on track. It gives me something to look forward to. I'd go crazy if I didn't have my Saturday night dinners out."

Mac, age 35, 58 pounds lost

Set the Scene for Success

Always eat in a calm atmosphere. Thriller movies, loud and fast music, and crowded places cause us to eat faster than we should. They also make us less aware of what we're eating. Always sit down when eating, and focus on the entire experience of eating. Try to taste and smell what you're eating to get the most out of it.

Think Thin

Using visualization seems to work in getting many dieters over the humps of a long-term diet. Here's how it works: Picture yourself at the weight you'd like to be, dressed in the clothes you've always wanted to wear, doing the things you've always wanted to do. Now picture how others will react to you at your new weight. Concentrate on the feelings these thoughts evoke.

15

"I try to spend five minutes after each meal just savoring the experience. I find that I enjoy the meal much more, and reach my satiety level."

Meg, age 44, 17 pounds lost

"I find if I talk a lot during my meal, I'm just not as satisfied. Sometimes I'm not even aware of what I ate, or how much I ate."

Rich, age 36, 20 pounds lost

"I have to put my fork down while I'm chewing, or I'll plow through much too quickly to enjoy what I'm eating."

Paul, age 49, 92 pounds lost

Yo Yo Dieting Is Not Dangerous

Even if you've been on a diet roller coaster for most of your life, it's less dangerous to your health to go up and down than it is to remain overweight. It doesn't hurt your metabolism, your cholesterol, or your blood pressure. It also doesn't make the pounds harder to budge.

"I can't believe that it took me seven tries to finally keep off that 40 pounds. Each time I tried, I would get within five pounds of my goal and gain it back. The first six times were expensive weight programs, all of which you'd recognize. Only when I made up my own plan was I able to get it off and keep it off, which I've done for ten years."

Linda, age 50, 40 pounds lost

Make Sure You're Ready

Now may not be the right time to diet if:

1. When food comes up in a conversation, on TV, etc., it makes you hungry even if you've just eaten.

2. While losing weight, you constantly fantasize about your favorite foods.

3. While losing weight, your mood is one of anger and deprivation.

4. You expect to lose more than 3 to 4 pounds a week.

5. You cannot differentiate between physical and emotional hunger.

"My trigger food is pistachio ice cream. It's the one food that I crave, and causes me to break my diet. So before I finally lost the weight, I allowed myself a week of all the pistachio ice cream I wanted. I had to get it out of my system."

Chandra, age 26, 14 pounds lost

Prepare Yourself

Some of the biggest challenges to dieters are the social situations that crop up in everyday life. It is not practical to try to hide away from these events, so what can you do? Not to worry—simply preparing yourself for dining out, parties, family gatherings, etc., can keep you from breaking your diet. Watch out for the hidden calories and too much alcohol. For every glass of an alcoholic beverage you drink, accompany it with a glass of ice water. This will keep you from becoming bloated, and will diffuse some of the effects. Choose fruit if you want dessert, or skip it altogether. If you do go off track, just get going again the next day.

"I always eat a light snack before I go to a party. Then I know I'll be in control when I get there."

Tammy, age 41, 13 pounds lost

"I wear the most body revealing outfit I can find. When I was overweight I would purposely pick something loose so that I had room to eat. Knowing that what I'm wearing will not allow for binging keeps me in line."

Tina, age 33, 75 pounds lost

17

"I used to think about all the delicious food that was waiting for me at that special event. Now I go for the people."

Nick, age 67, 38 pounds lost

"My problem was the vending machine at the office. Now I make certain to bring a bag of carrots, and keep it right on top of my desk."

Wendy, age 32, 28 pounds lost

Seek Support

Find someone in your life you can commiserate with a least once a day. Feeling isolated can cause even the most determined dieter to fall off.

"I found a friend on the Internet who had a similar weight problem. We compared notes daily. Just writing to her made me feel better."

Polly, age 35, 68 pounds lost

"Making myself accountable to someone was as good for me as going to an expensive diet program. At the end of each day, I called a friend who was known for her disciplined lifestyle and not only did she encourage me, but always had a new tip for my next day's challenge."

Sandy, age 25, 13 pounds lost

Organize Yourself

Too much free time on your hands can very often lead to mindless eating. On a sheet of paper, write out a daily schedule. Map out the time (in the beginning you'll need to do this by the half hour) and try to sneak in some activity. Note the dangerous spots of the day. For instance, if you tend to snack while waiting for dinner to cook, turn on the radio and dance around!

Count It Out

Silly as it sounds, this secret seems to work when you're enticed to reach for that tempting snack. Before you dig into that carton of ice cream, cookie bag, etc., take a deep breath and count to 100. Usually, by the time you stop counting you will have convinced yourself that you don't really need it.

Use Lists

Shop with a list and you'll be less likely to compulsively pick things out, and end up with fattening goodies that will sabotage your efforts. You'll only gain a more expensive grocery tab, and you'll be missing things you need to keep on track.

Push Yourself

Only you can get yourself off the couch to exercise, cook that healthy dish, and move that body.

Why We Diet

67 percent to be healthier

21 percent to look better

6 percent for a better love life

3 percent for a better job

3 percent just don't know

—from a survey by Johns Hopkins University

Maximize Your Breathing

The way you breathe can give you energy that you thought could only come from food. Many of us breathe shallowly through our mouths, which actually saps energy and keeps our body in a state of stress. Taking deep, slow, controlled breaths through your nose will get more air into your lungs and bloodstream. This will also cause waste products to be taken out of your body tissues more efficiently.

Don't Expect Too Much

Strange, isn't it, that we always want it all—and right now. Make certain that your expectations are reasonable. Expect to feel healthier, look better, and be more fabulous than you've ever been. If you expect that first, before expecting to reach that low mark on the scale, you're more likely to actually achieve it all.

"Deciding to let destiny guide my final outcome was a real 'freeing' experience for me. I made the decision to only put food into my body that would nurture it and help it run more efficiently. I let my body figure out what my weight should be, not some dumb chart."

Eva, age 34, 66 pounds lost

Learn to Enjoy Life

Get beyond the idea that your life is all about your weight and food. While you're losing weight, gain the pleasures of those physical, spiritual, and intellectual components that make you fully human.

Break Some Rules

Yes, most diets don't call for cookies. But if a cookie a day makes you feel like one of the living, go for it. It's your life, your body, and only you know what you need to get you through the day. Just remember that while one cookie is fine, a whole bag will make you feel worse.

Chapter Two

Dieting Myths

Diet Supplements

You already know by now how dangerous prescription weight loss supplements can be. Many over-the-counter supplements, if used inappropriately, can cause dizziness and other side effects.

Food Fakes

Frozen Yogurt: Has less calcium and as much sugar as regular yogurt, without the benefits of active cultures.

Sports Drinks: These highly acidic beverages contain lots of calories and can harm tooth enamel.

Fat-Free Pretzels: Don't bother—pretzels are already low in fat.

Low Fat Cookies: You'll end up eating too many, because the truth is they just don't satisfy.

Unrealistic Goals

Don't set yourself up for failure. You'll sabotage all your good efforts if you compare yourself to airbrushed models or professionally made-up movie stars.

Forgetting Calories

Believing the latest hype that it's fat grams that count, many dieters have found the weight just not moving, because they don't look at the calorie count of what they're eating. Remember, it's a combination of the two that will get you to your goal.

Money Doesn't Buy Motivation

Dieters have been fooled into spending large sums of money to enter a diet club or program that promises to help you lose the weight. Remember, you are still the one doing the work, no matter how much you spend on some pricey gimmick.

"I became a diet club junkie, going from program to program. I'm sure that I spent thousands of dollars, believing that someone else was going to set me free from my years of overeating. It was only when I came to the decision to take charge of my own body that I dropped the pounds."

Dan, age 47, 130 pounds lost

"Boy, was I in the wrong place. I had only 15 pounds to lose, so I thought I would go to a weekly weigh-in to keep me honest. The lecturer was 25 pounds heavier than me, and then had the nerve to give me a goal that was totally unrealistic."

Sue, age 31, 16 pounds lost

Fasting

Although some dieters have had success with a one day a week fruit "detox" diet, most reported that fasting only caused lightheadedness and deep feelings of deprivation.

Low Self-Esteem

A report by the University of Wisconsin-Madison cites that men and women with low self-esteem were more likely to be overweight, smoke, consume more alcohol, and expose themselves to dangerous situations.

"While losing the weight, I went into therapy. I realized I needed to fix my head while working on my body."

Marcie, age 28, 47 pounds lost

Believing Setbacks Are Fatal

Learning to accept setbacks as a part of being human will help you cause yourself less frustration on the road to success. Setbacks, when viewed as learning tools, actually help dieters achieve their final goals. Just about every person with a great body I've encountered has experienced a glitch somewhere in their attempt to slim down. Those who succeeded were able to step back, analyze what went wrong, correct the problem(s), and then use it as part of their motivation.

"When I started the final program that became my final success, I took pen in hand and listed all the times I had tried to lose weight in my life, and what happened that made me get off track. What I found was that it was the same situation playing itself over and over again."

Chandra, age 51, 58 pounds lost

Not Setting Goals

Failure to set goals and a time table throws the whole diet experience up in the air. While unrealistic goal setting (ten pounds in one week, five dress sizes by that reunion, etc.) can sabotage even the most determined dieter, there has to be some sort of pot at the end of the rainbow. Maybe your goal will be to drop a size by your birthday or learn a healthy way to fix your favorite dish. Make it a goal that will eventually get you to your long-awaited success.

"I found that mapping out a goal that had nothing and everything to do with my weight loss was an important key in getting me back to the old me that I had lost. At the end of every month, I called an old friend. My weight had made me embarrassed to be seen, and as the weight came off, so did my shame."

Buck, age 42, 155 pounds lost

Fear of Judgment
Some dieters wouldn't leave their homes because they were so ashamed of their weight gain. They created a "Catch-22" situation—with the world revolving around them, they would sit home, consoling themselves with ice cream, chips, etc.

"While my girlfriends would go out on dates, I would stay home, sit on my couch and cry into my Chinese take out. Saturday nights were brutal! Becoming my own best friend, going to movies by myself (the biggest milestone), shopping alone, and seeking out others who were also 'dateless' took me out of my self-pitying mode that made things feel so much worse."

Felicia, age 25, 57 pounds lost

Bad Habits
List all those bad habits and change them into good ones.

"Believe me, I never thought that cleaning my plate was a bad habit, but when I was really full, I would continue to eat until everything was gone.

24

Leaving food on my plate was hard to do, but helped me get my appetite back in check. But even today, I occasionally can hear my mother telling me about all the starving children who would be happy to have my food. Sorry, Mom, but it never made me happy to hear that."

Cassie, age 45, 69 pounds lost

Using Food to Rebuild Energy

Why is it when people are tired, they believe that only food will get them going again? The problem is that it's not so much that they eat, it's the foods they're choosing. Eating regularly is one of the best ways to keep energy high and fuel metabolic processes. However, choosing junk food as a quick fix will cause brain sugar to rise suddenly and then crash. It's a temporary fix that generally lasts no longer than an hour. While it's tempting to reach for a chocolate bar, fruit is absorbed more slowly

Putting Yourself First

Believing that spending time on yourself is too self-indulgent only leads you on the road to failure. Taking time to become the best you can be allows you to give to others and feel good about doing it.

25

into the body and will provide an even energy boost without the highs and lows of sugary snacks.

Here's another idea. When you get tired, rest! A cat nap is a no-calorie revitalizer!

Not Understanding the Dynamics

The truth is that there are reasons lurking behind many weight problems. Yes, there are genetic components and family customs that may be responsible, but there also may be hidden sexual or physical abuse and other issues that no diet can cure. There is no diet that can cure emotional pain. Understanding this, perhaps including professional therapy, might be necessary before the real transformation can begin.

Refusing to Grow Up

Food cravings can be reminders of our childhood.

Comfort foods are usually the foods that Mom made for you when you came home and it was cold, the school bully caught up with you, etc. These foods still feel good today. Researchers have found that it isn't just taste, but the chemical reaction to the brain that makes these foods so appealing.

Believing It's Glandular

In only a very few instances is it true that weight problems are caused by the glands. But if this thinking is holding you back, go check it out with a doctor. Either way, you'll then be able to get on with a solution.

Limiting Cereals and Breads

Many believe that eliminating cereals and breads from their diet would help them achieve their goals. But the fact is that there's no one food that's bad for you. It's always a matter of quantity.

"I happen to adore bread. I love baking it, checking out ethnic bakeries, and the smell is heavenly! I also believe it's been a major player in my ongoing struggles with weight. I knew I'd never make it down the scale without bread. I kept it in my diet, but rather than slathering it in butter, jams, etc., I decided to eat the bread, and nothing else. I limited myself to two slices a day, and I made sure that I microwaved it. This way, the replete, just-baked taste made me feel absolutely decadent."

Maura, age 36, 32 pounds lost

"Sometimes I make cereal my supper. I like the fun of eating cereal, the fiber is good for me, and it usually is fairly high in protein. It has been essential in helping me with my final weight loss.

Adding fruit makes it a complete meal."

Sue, age 27, 19 pounds lost

"I look for the low fat breads now available at most natural supermarkets. They are surprisingly tasty, and contain lots of nutrients. Bread seems to calm me down and keep me feeling satisfied."

Mandy, age 33, 20 pounds lost

Bananas Are Fattening

Although a banana is sweeter than an apple or orange, it has only 85 calories. Bananas are a wonderful source of potassium and contain valuable protein. Dieters report bananas are more filling than some of the other fruits, and they're also great for alleviating constipation.

Exercising Is Dangerous During a Menstrual Cycle

Actually, women who exercise during their periods find that it helps to alleviate their cramps. Of course, it's important to listen to your body and only do what your body can.

Vitamins Give You Energy

There are a lot of people popping vitamins in the morning, believing that they're getting an energy boost for the day. The fact is that the energy you get is from the nutrients in the foods you eat. That's why it is important to put foods into your body that will provide you with the proper fuel to get through your day. Especially when you're dieting, it is important to choose foods which will provide the most power. But since you are most likely cutting down on what you eat, some supplementation is not a bad idea.

Chicken and Fish Are Lower in Cholesterol

The cholesterol content in chicken and fish is virtually the same as in other meats. However, poultry and fish do have a lower fat content than most red meat.

Losing Five Pounds Is No Big Deal

Oh, yeah? Take a five pound bag of sugar and carry it around for an hour. Then you'll begin to appreciate those minor milestones of your weight loss. Every bit of weight you lose brings improved health and vitality.

Carbohydrates Make You Fat

Lately, just about every article or book around blames carbohydrates for all the problems of extra weight. Why blame carbohydrates? Because reducing fat and calories didn't work. Neither did reducing protein. So what else is left to blame? The truth is that researchers have found some serious problems with the oh-so-trendy high protein diets of late. There is evidence that these diets are not very healthy and may lead to certain medical conditions. Plus, researchers point out that not all carbohydrates are the same.

Low Fat Foods Are Low in Sugar

This myth has really helped the fat-free cookie market. Unfortunately it's just not true. Simply because a food is low fat, doesn't mean it's necessarily healthy. These low fat foods may be loaded with sugar, sodium, and chemical preservatives.

Natural Vitamins Are Better

Not only is this not true, but most of the time your body can't tell the difference between a vitamin from food or a test tube. In fact, scientists find that some "natural" vitamin sources contain higher

Standing Up to Eat Will Burn More Calories

Not only is this dieting myth not true, but eating like this will cause you to overeat. You should never eat when standing up unless absolutely necessary.

levels of contaminants than more carefully refined ingredients used in the manufacturing process.

Grilled Vegetables Are Lower in Calories

The next time you're in a restaurant, I hope you will watch how grilled vegetables are cooked. They throw so much oil on them that the vegetables, especially the soft ones (zucchini, eggplant, mushrooms, etc.), just soak it up. This turns that grilled veggie dish into one of the heaviest entrees listed on a restaurant's menu!

Earrings to Control Cravings

There are a host of "magnetic wellness" products, one of which is an earring that allegedly controls appetite and cravings. The earrings supposedly work on the same premise as acupuncture. A part of the ear is related to hunger, and the earrings

press on that spot to stop cravings. Quite a few of the more "desperate dieters" have tried these peculiar posts, and the only thing that stopped them from eating was that the pain they experienced wearing these earrings made it impossible to concentrate on anything else.

Subliminal Tapes

Lots of companies have come out with motivational tapes to lose weight. Success levels with them are questionable. In fact, one of my interviewees said that the voice on the tape was so annoying that the stress from listening to him drove her to the refrigerator.

Be Wary of Mr. Muffin Man

Muffins are as different as Olympians and couch potatoes. While some are fairly healthy, like oat bran, others contain as many as 450 calories. Not only is it important to look for low fat muffins and muffins rich in fiber, but also be sure to check calorie content. Some low fat muffins contain as many calories as regular muffins because of added sugar.

Brown Sugar Is Better Than White
All brown sugar has over its white counterpart is a little bit of molasses. It is not nutritionally superior.

Spot Exercise Can Reduce Fatty Areas
While spot exercising can tighten muscle, it has no effect on fat.

Exercising in Special Sweats and Rubber Aids Fat Elimination
It seems to appear to work because you lose water through perspiration. However, the body will hang on to the fat, and the weight will come right back.

Margarine Is Better Than Butter
Here's the truth. Margarine is completely man-made and has absolutely no nutritional benefits. Butter is natural and has anti-cancer and anti-viral properties. There is research in its early stages that says butter may even help in the prevention and treatment of Alzheimer's disease. Unfortunately, some margarine has been linked with causing cancer. Butter contains the same amount of fat as margarine. Margarine's only benefit is that it contains no cholesterol, while butter contains about 12 grams per tablespoon. So do spread it sparingly.

Eliminate Eggs
Don't bother! Eggs have always been good for you. Eating eggs a couple of times a week as an

entree will give you an excellent protein meal with few calories. Load up that omelet with lots of vegetables as a delicious diet tool.

Microwaves Destroy Vitamins

The opposite is true. Less vitamins are destroyed this way than in traditional ovens. Microwaves pass through your food without any harmful effects.

Nonfat Foods Are Healthiest

This is another long-held myth that has held us hostage from food enjoyment. Fat in food not only curbs hunger, but it helps keep insulin levels steady.

Caffeinated Beverages Can Energize

These popular drinks have a dehydrating effect that can drain your energy. Coffee, tea, and soda are stimulants that bring you up quickly and then let you crash. It's important when drinking any caffeinated beverage to chase it with an equal amount of ice water. It's also important to drink water with every alcoholic beverage, another dehydrator.

Saunas Can Help Shed Pounds

Although sitting in a sauna can feel great, any weight you lose is water weight. Once you replenish the fluids you've lost, the weight comes right back.

Fasting Eliminates Toxins

Each and every scientist I interviewed refuted any evidence that fasting eliminates toxins of any variety. Do it for religious reasons or to protest nuclear waste sites, but your body naturally eliminates unwanted substances through the usual waste processes.

Form Doesn't Matter When Exercising

Weight training and cardiovascular workouts can backfire if you're doing them wrong because you may end up working a different muscle than intended. Worse, you can put unnecessary stress on your joints.

"I thought I would try to exercise from some charts I found in a magazine. I ended up doing it wrong, and bulked up in the area I had hoped to slim."

Jerry, age 25, 32 pounds lost

Taste Bud Inhibitor

This is an orthodontically fitted mouth piece that covers the taste buds on the roof of your mouth so that you can't enjoy the taste of food. It costs about $300.00 and requires a dentist to fit it properly. Save your money. Taste is not the only reason we eat.

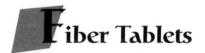

Fiber Tablets

The problem with these tablets is that they don't provide the variety of fiber that you get with natural fiber. If you're looking for a fiber supplement to add to your diet, try the liquid fiber supplements available at most drugstores. Better yet, choose a breakfast cereal with at least six grams of fiber. That should do it.

33

Corsets for Weight Contouring

Women all over the country are picking up on the new undergarments that hearken back to the Victorian era. Today's corsets allege to celebrate the female form, when in fact they are reviving the barbaric practices of the past. Some women are corseting themselves as a way to control their eating. They can only digest fruits and grains—pizza would be prohibitive. Physicians report that some of the dangers of corseting include muscle atrophy (the body stops relying on natural muscle), aching kidneys, digestive problems, and unhealthy pressure on the organs. It can also interrupt breathing and even hinder menstrual cycles.

Lack of Time

With grocery aisles full of healthy packaged foods, it can't get much easier, no matter how little time you have to cook, to stay on track with your diet. Make up your menus ahead of time, and stock up on low fat packaged foods so when you come home stressed out, wanting that quick fix, you'll have a variety of meals ready to cater to your taste at the time. Ideally you should be able to combine a packaged food with something fresh. Happily, fresh foods are also becoming more convenient, like cut-up salad mixes. Meat also comes cut-up, and vegetables now come peeled and sliced too. And don't forget breakfast foods for a quick, satisfying meal anytime of day.

Alcohol and Diets Don't Mix

Although alcohol contains calories, there are low calorie choices. Champagne and wine spritzers top the list. If your lifestyle has always allowed for social drinking, there is no reason to stop. Just stay away from the eggnog and that occasional drink will blend right into your weight loss efforts. According to the American Cancer Society, active women who walked at least four hours a week, ate a vegetable-rich diet, and had a glass of wine or beer with dinner up to five nights a week lost more abdominal weight than healthy, active nondrinkers.

Overdoing and Rushing Your Program

You'll burn out faster than a match in a wind tunnel if you try to do it all at once. Not only that, you could cause yourself serious health damage short- and long-term.

The Diet Shot

Some alternative diet doctors are administering injections of adrenal cortex extract. The highly controversial extract is taken from the adrenal glands of cattle, sheep, and other animals. The concept is that the injection will help ease a dieter's salt cravings and regulate their blood pressure. There is no research proving these benefits, and there have been bacterial infections involved. The Food and Drug Administration has issued alerts and warnings of serious, life-threatening injuries associated with such shots.

Trying to Look Like Barbie, Today's Supermodels, and Mannequins

Yes, there are some women who are having plastic surgery to look like this physically impossible childhood creature, but it just can't be done. Not only are Barbie's vital statistics physiologically impossible, her neck is twice the length of that of a normal human being.

The typical model weighs 20 percent less than the average woman. Just ten years ago, she weighed 8 to 10 percent less.

The vital statistics of store mannequins are so extreme that if a woman tried to equate their shape, she would not have enough body fat to menstruate.

Fast Music Eating

Listening to your favorite dance tune while you're eating will get your mouth moving and plate clean in record time. There have been numerous studies that suggest that people who listen to fast music while dining will take more and larger forkfuls of food per minute than those who listen to slow music. Those doo-wopping diners took an average five forkfuls per minute while the slow dancers, or no-music diners, took only three. The fast music diners also were more apt to ask for seconds. The reason you need to slow your eating down is that the brain needs to register that it's full, and once it does, you consume less.

Bright Colors

"Hot" colors, including red, orange, and yellow, stimulate your mood and your appetite. That's bad news if you're trying to cut down. That's why McDonald's (yellow arches) and other fast food chains use these colors to their advantage. Make certain that the dishes you use are either clear, white, or pastel, and that your dining area is decorated in soft tones.

Boredom

Make sure that there's enough variety in your diet, workouts, and your life. More dieters went off their diets because of the sheer tedium than for any other reason.

Too Little Calories

Consume enough to fuel your body, but not so many that they get stored as fat. Skip "empty" calories with no nutritional value.

Energy Bars

Only use these convenience bars in an emergency. Don't use them as meal replacements. They contain too many calories for the little satisfaction that they provide. They really are intended for professional athletes, and somehow have made their way over to the diet population.

Skipping Breakfast

Your body has been on an 8 to 12 hour fast. It needs fuel. You'll only make up for it later.

"I never made time for breakfast, and I was always first at the morning coffee line, picking up that jelly doughnut."

Frank, age 45, 53 pounds lost

Basing Worth on Weight

Feeling that you need to be the skinniest belle of the ball may mean that you have serious esteem issues that no diet can cure.

"Every morning my mood would be decided by my weight. If I was a pound or two down, I was absolutely up, on a real high. If the scale showed a higher number than the previous day, I was impossible to be around. I finally had to throw away my scale until I got myself straight. Now, I've reincorporated the scale into my weight management, but I only allow myself to use it once a week."

Vicki, age 38, 45 pounds lost

37

Chapter Three

Tricks and Tools

Keeping Out of the Frig

How can you keep from opening the refrigerator the average of 22 times a day?

1. Stay hydrated by drinking water and low calorie beverages each hour. What we often think is hunger is sometimes thirst.

2. Take a walk (around the block, in the yard, etc.) for 15 minutes. Sometimes it's just boredom or an emotional need you're feeling.

3. Lie down for a few minutes. You may be tired and need a few minutes to restore your energy.

Write a Note to Yourself

Write a letter to yourself listing all the reasons you are finally ready to lose weight. Keep this letter with you at all times and look at it from time to time. Whenever you feel yourself getting out of control, let it inspire you to keep going.

Drink Ice Water

The body burns up to 40 negative calories just by turning up its metabolism in order to warm the water.

Stop the Love Affair with Food

Call a friend when you feel lonely. Food can never be a companion.

Food Is Fuel

Just as you want the highest quality gas for your car, you must choose foods that best maintain your energy and keep your metabolism working, as well as satisfying your palate. Choose carefully. Your body doesn't deserve "junk."

Garbage Foods

Throw garbage foods away and simplify your life and diet with the best quality foods you can afford. They do nothing to help, and look at the harm they've done.

Eat Often

Eating multiple small meals a day may work better for you than eating fewer larger ones, especially if you are first embarking on a diet and trying to get over the constant "hungries."

When dieting, your body first loses fat from the areas you last put it on.

Sit Down!

Absolutely do not take a bite unless you're sitting down in the kitchen or dining room. Do not wander around the house with a trail of goodies, and don't eat in front of the TV.

Laugh It Up!

Researchers have found that just one good belly laugh is worth 5 minutes on the treadmill.

Retrain Your Taste Buds

If your past weight loss programs have failed due to boredom, flavor up those low calorie foods by exploring the hundreds of herbs that are now available in both fresh and dried form. Fat is an acquired taste. You can retrain your palate with fat-free flavors.

Pinch Your Ear, Lose Your Appetite

Reflexologists advise that pinching your ear will curb cravings and lessen the appetite. Apply pressure with clean hands, one at a time, to the front of the ear. This is the area that affects hunger.

Read Labels

Check out the fat, fiber, and calorie content. It only takes a few seconds and could make all the difference in your success.

Enjoy the Compliment

When people compliment you on your weight loss, they are telling you that they respect the effort and challenge you've met. Believe them!

Do It One Day at a Time

Anything other than one day at a time is too overwhelming and self defeating. It's the motto of Alcoholics Anonymous, and there is a definite commonality.

Slow Down

You'll enjoy your food more, eat less of it, and the chewing will relieve stress.

Looks Aren't Everything

It may look great on the plate, but how will it look on you?

Start a Piggy Bank

Put the money that you would spend in the vending machine, at the bakery, etc., into a new clothes fund. That small change can add up quickly.

Check Your Head

Never eat anything bigger than your head, even lettuce. You'll only stretch your stomach out. Train your tummy to settle for less.

Big Isn't Better

When it comes to your favorite high fat foods, buy the smallest container available. Eat it, get it out of your system, and then get it out of the house.

Check Out Supermarket Carts

Supermarket carts tell you a lot about the person driving them. Take a look at what other people have in their carts at the grocery store. Now check yours. Are there any items you are embarrassed about checking out or having someone see? Then put it back.

Who's the Boss?

Since when do you take orders from a doughnut? You are in control.

Goodies?

If they're so "good" why do they make you unhappy, overweight, and unable to get into your clothes?

Say "No"

If you find you're just too darn polite to say "no," then say "no thank you."

Create a Chart

Take a piece of graph paper and mark your daily progress. Attach a reward at the end of each 5 or 10 pound interval.

Weigh Your Portions

A small, inexpensive diet scale will become a teaching tool until you can learn to measure by "eye."

Brush Your Tongue and Teeth

After you finish a meal, or when you feel like snacking, brush your teeth and your tongue. Use a minty toothpaste. Sometimes when we think we want to eat, we just want to get that nasty taste out of our mouths. The fresh taste will curb your desire. You won't want to ruin that fresh feeling.

Record Your Measurements

Just as important as your weight, keep track of your measurements weekly. The tape measure will show true progress even when the scale isn't moving. Sometimes excess water, salt, etc., can give a false weight gain.

43

Keep Your Breath Sweet

Sugar-free breath mints are a dieter's ally. It's a calorie bargain at about 3 calories a mint.

Create a Snacking Budget

Allow yourself 200 calories a day for snacks. Make a list and deduct from it as you go through your day. The list can include popcorn, sugar-free Jell-O, salsa, etc.

Take a Deep Breath

It may sound too simplistic, but the International Breath Institute swears that oxygen is one of the keys to losing weight. Focus on breathing deeply, into your stomach, not just your chest. When you breathe in, try to exhale longer than you inhale. This will eliminate toxins that will otherwise be stored as fat.

Get Over the Defiance

Some dieters who went into therapy over their weight problems traced their issues back to eating to defy others' expectations. These dieters were the typical "secret" eaters.

"I discovered that weight clubs were not the answer for me. The counselors would make me feel 'good' or 'bad,' just like a child. I found myself going back home and eating anything that stood still just for spite."

Pat, age 34, 40 pounds lost

Have an Alternative Plan

Whether it's a behavior or a food, there should always be an alternative. All or nothing doesn't work in the real world. If your downfall is something crisp, keep low-fat crispy products on hand, like popcorn or rice cakes. If you get caught up in a TV program, have a stair stepper, treadmill, or even a jump rope in the room.

Smell the Coffee

Research suggests that certain smells can trick the brain into thinking that the stomach is full. The aroma of coffee (especially flavored), peppermint, and even green apple can help. Whatever you choose to eat, incorporate the aromatic benefits of smell.

Do It Naturally

Add fresh fruits and vegetables to your diet whenever you can. Use the produce aisle as your primary snacking aisle. Fruits and vegetables are high in fiber and will help you feel more full.

Paint It Black

You'll eat less on a black or navy blue plate.

Sleep for Weight Loss

Suffering from sleep deprivation can cause you to snack unnecessarily (usually with comfort foods).

Warm It Up

Serve yourself up some warm bread and you'll find you really don't need butter. Steam up some vegetables, and they'll be more satisfying than a cold salad. Plus, the food aromas will help satisfy the brain.

Eat Your Sweets at Breakfast

Your body is at optimal calorie burning mode in the morning. So if you can't go through the day without that little treat, you'll burn it off more efficiently if you have it in the morning. Our metabolisms are naturally speedier during the day when we're more active.

Turn Up the Air

Try to keep your room a little chilly at night. The more heat your body needs, the more calories you'll burn to provide that heat.

Save the Packaging

If you love a certain food, save the wrapper even after you've eaten it. Smell it when you're hungry. You'll trick yourself into believing you ate it. Models buy candy bars, throw away the candy, and carry the wrappers in their model's bag.

Don't Swallow!

Models and other successful bodies are also known for taking a forbidden bite, chewing, and spitting it out.

Alcohol Weakens Willpower

Always alternate alcoholic drinks with water. Offer to be the designated driver to cement your commitment.

Cut the Fat

Take as much fat off as you can before you cook meat and chicken. And don't even think about keeping the skin!

Perfume Replaces Chocolate

When a chocolate craving comes your way, take a whiff of a strong perfume. Carry a full strength perfume with you, or perfume a hanky. Put it up to your nose when you pass a bakery.

Wear a Belt

Find a belt that fits too snugly to be comfortable. Try to wear it to keep you aware of why you need to diet. If you just can't wear it, at least try it on once a week to watch the inches fall away.

Find a Friend

Studies have found that friends push each other in a way that causes them to lose weight 20 percent faster than if they tried to do it alone. This friendly push helps with both diet and exercise.

Become a Little Selfish

Don't waste the energy you need to be successful by getting caught up in someone else's drama of life. Don't put yourself last.

Out of Sight, Out of Mind

If you lack any semblance of willpower, just don't bring the things that cause you weakness in the house. If you must bake, freeze the extras or give them away.

Eat More Colorfully

The deeper the color, the more powerful the cancer and disease fighting antioxidants. Choose red grapes over green, and Romaine lettuce over iceberg. Dieters also report that the deeper colors have more taste.

Lower the Heat

When cooking, lowering the heat requires using less oil or shortening.

Change Your Route

If you enter your house through the kitchen door and can't get by the refrigerator without stopping, then change your route. Don't walk by the vending machine or doughnut cart at work. If you are greatly affected by TV commercials, get up or start reading while they're on.

Drink Something Warm

Warm liquids give your stomach a feeling of fullness. Dieters report satisfaction from bouillon, tea, and flavored coffees (sugarless).

Waiting Is Control

Sometimes just the smell or sight of food can take even the most resolute dieter off track. The best defense is to distract yourself for ten minutes. Walk away if you have to. The urge usually disappears.

Give in Just a Little

If you really must have a particular food, purchase one portion, not the whole bag, and certainly not the big bargain size. If you want ice cream, buy a small sized cone. Hungry for fries? Choose the small bag. The scale won't even notice these small splurges.

Track Your Triggers

Write down every moment you experience a lapse in judgment. What were you feeling at the time? Who were you with at the time? When and how did it occur?

48

Deal with It

A demanding boss, abusive relationship, or loneliness can't be cured with food. Find a new career, go into counseling, and do something besides stuffing your mouth to change your situation. Choose nonfood strategies to alleviate your problems.

Make a Bet

Putting your money where your mouth is by betting that you will lose a certain amount of weight with a coworker, friend, relative, or enemy will be more inspirational to losing those pounds.

Make It Beautiful

Food should look as great as it tastes in order to provide total satisfaction. Making each meal an event will make even the most meager portions inviting. It's the secret of the dining experience known as "nouvelle cuisine." Use it in your own kitchen.

Seduction

Remove temptation from the kitchen counter (cookie jar, etc.) and replace it with a creative fruit bowl.

Don't Settle for Less

Track when your cravings usually occur and have a snack ready to go just before they usually strike.

Enjoy Your Life

Improve upon your favorite things. If you have your favorite programs, use them to your advantage. Buy a stationary bicycle, treadmill, or inexpensive stair stepper. Position it right by the TV, and time your workouts to coincide with your "can't miss it" shows. Get into your show and watch the time fly by.

"I love going out with my coworkers every Friday evening. Was I about to end this enjoyable ritual?

No way! I had to come up with a way to join them in every way but the food. While they're ordering appetizers, I choose a clear consommé. When they go for the entree, I choose an appetizer. I even have dessert with them, but mine is usually fruit."

Tina, age 35, 48 pounds lost

Count the Perks

Visualize all the ways your life will change for the better with a slimmer, healthier body. You'll finally find clothes that fit and flatter, you'll be able to participate in more family activities, and you'll have all that new energy. Did I mention all that extra time that you won't waste thinking about food?

Find the Passion

Think about that one thing you've always wanted to do, then go do it. It could be a new hobby, a career change, or tracing your family roots. A new focus will not only take your mind off food, but will create a positive feeling about what you're doing.

Not Everyone Has Your Best Interest in Mind

Sometimes friends and family will try to sabotage you and your diet plans. You'd better be ready for it. Far beyond "oh, just one won't hurt" will come "you should have started earlier," "I've known you too long," or "come on, you'll never get into that outfit by Friday." Most successful dieters handle these situations without becoming confrontational by directly asking for support. This puts some of the responsibility (and guilt) back on those friends.

"I lost a couple of friends because they wouldn't change to a restaurant with lower fat alternatives. I had to question, were they really that inflexible, or were they afraid that I would reach my goal?"

Sara, age 23, 28 pounds lost

Find Your Strength

Through each success you have on your diet, not only will you find the strength within yourself, you'll start to feel like you can move mountains (or at least that couch).

A Little Envy Is a Good Thing

Don't go crazy, but pick out someone who you'd like to look better than. Even better, imagine becoming that someone of whom others are envious. Competition is a great mobilizer. You can use this need to compete in a more positive way, like joining a walkathon (makes you feel good inside and out).

The Naked Truth

Once a day (morning or evening) take absolutely everything off, and look at yourself in a full length mirror. You'll be inspired to keep going. You'll see new muscle, a flatter stomach, and a new you emerging. Seeing yourself this way will be more revealing than any scale.

Check Your Relationship

Stress is the leading cause of weight gain. Studies indicate that couples overeat after a fight, and there's an average weight gain of twenty to thirty pounds after a divorce.

Get a Dog

If you don't have a Fido in the house, get one. Just as "in your face" as a personal trainer, he needs to be exercised and he's not allowed to go by himself. He'll keep at you until you take him out. Animals also encourage touch and contact, which relaxes the body, and lowers blood pressure.

Take a Few Bites

If you must have that sweet, just take a couple bites. A taste is what you want. The calories are not what you need.

Act Like a Grown-up

Eating food with a sophisticated flair will reeducate your taste buds into believing less is more.

Gaze into the Future

Foresee your life as a slimmer, healthier you. Keep brochures of that vacation you'll take, and keep mail order catalogs around of the great things you'll wear.

Commiserate

Call someone up who's trying to make their life better. It doesn't have to be a friend who's battling with their weight. It could be a colleague having work problems, a sister who's trying to stop smoking, a cousin who's trying to work out that gambling problem. It helps to know that we're not alone.

Know Your Limit

To calculate the maximum calories you can eat and still lose weight, simply add a zero to your current weight. For example, someone who weighs 130 pounds can eat up to 1,300 calories a day and still lose weight.

Sit Up Straight

You'll burn at least ten percent more calories sitting upright than reclining. So try to sit up when you're reading or watching TV. Good posture when standing also burns more calories than slouching.

Restrict Your Choices

There have been several studies done recently which prove that the more food choices we have, the more we eat. There was even a study that showed that we eat more with a plate of differently shaped pasta than with a single shaped pasta.

Finish Off with Floss

Brush and floss immediately after meals to discourage snacking.

Hitting a Plateau Is Not Failure

Don't lose your motivation when you seem to hit a plateau on your diet—it will pass. Sometimes we get impatient and go off our diet when we level off for a time. But don't worry, just coast for as long as you need to.

Buy the Best

Buy the freshest, highest quality food you can afford. Depriving yourself of good food sets yourself up for failure. If you enjoy the foods on your diet, you'll be more likely to stick to it.

53

Switch Meals Around

If you're dying for pizza at 8 a.m., eat it for breakfast. Otherwise, you'll just overeat on other things, and still eat the pizza (probably the whole pie) at night. Get the craving out of your system.

Dim the Lights

Before sitting down to eat, try turning down the lights. Johns Hopkins University reports that people reduce their appetite when dining under low lighting. Bright lights stimulate us psychologically. If you don't have dimming lights, then try candles.

Stop the Love Affair with Food

Connect with people when you're feeling lonely. Just getting away from yourself will help keep you from getting out of control.

Satisfy Your Sweet Tooth

Your sweet tooth will not leave you alone, so you might as well give in. Look, a butterscotch candy has only 25 calories, lasts about fifteen minutes in your mouth, and tastes absolutely sinful. Go for it.

Don't Hate Her Because She's Thin

It's not fair to malign people just because they're slim. While some people stay thin no matter how much ice cream they inhale, the majority of us gain weight even thinking about something sinful. Blame your metabolism. You will never have this luxury, so you might as well face up to it.

Run Away

Sometimes there is just nothing you can do when food calls your name. That's when you have to run out of the house or leave the office—just go. Even if it's just to walk around the block, you're getting away from that call of food can become so compelling. Go clear your head. It might just save your diet.

Spirituality May Help

Some of the successful dieters I interviewed found that it was only when they turned to a higher power that they were able to finally lick the demon of excess weight. It has helped many in twelve step programs, and is the basis for Overeaters Anonymous.

"It was only when I regained my childhood faith that I was able to turn off the voices in my head that kept me from reaching my goal. I don't know where they were coming from, but prayer kept them away."

Phil, age 43, 90 pounds lost

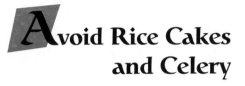

Avoid Rice Cakes and Celery

There is no way you can succeed if you try to maintain a diet with the foods you avoid when you're not dieting. When you're suffering through a diet, you have no energy, you're bored, and you'll look terrible. You (and anyone who sees you) will wonder why you even bothered.

Divide Your Plate

You need to watch your nutrients, and the easiest way is to divide your plate into four quarters. Fill three-quarters with vegetables and fruit, and one quarter with beans, meat, or dairy.

Learn to Measure Food with Your Eye

A serving of rice is the size of your fist. A one ounce serving of cheese is about the size of your thumb. A serving of meat is about the size of a deck of cards. Dieters are usually shocked to find out how small a "one serving" really is.

Save Time

If a recipe, exercise, or healthy habit takes too much time, it won't last in your routine. Strip it back, or eliminate it completely, and find something easier to take its place. Streamlining our activities will allow them to become lifetime habits. Our society is full speed ahead, and our diets must fit in.

Watch Out for the Calorie Creep

Unnoticed calories creep in when you're most relaxed. When you're dining with friends and family, you can easily consume up to 800 calories and not even realize it. Sharing dishes and bottles of wine are both dangerous habits, making portion control virtually impossible. Without looking too "Grinch-like," measure out your portions, dip in only once, and drink lots of water while everyone else is digging in.

Chapter Four

Food Choices

You Should Eat

First, the good news. Severe rationing of calories in a diet makes it harder, rather than easier, to lose weight. Dieters who eat more of low fat foods lose weight more efficiently than those who eat lower calorie menus with more fat. Eating the right foods can actually boost your body's ability to burn fat. Also, studies done on drastic weight loss programs have proven that decreased brain function and reaction time are consequences of such a dramatic change.

What Should I Eat?

Topping your list of foods to include on your diet should be those that stimulate the body to lose weight. These include:

Grains: pasta, oatmeal, corn, pretzels, popcorn, rice

Fruits: apples, cherries, oranges, grapefruit, bananas

Vegetables: broccoli, spinach, carrots, green beans

Great Munchies

Don't think twice about these snacks. You can munch away and still lose the pounds. With these foods, you almost burn more calories chewing and digesting them than they actually contain.

Under 20 Calories

1 cup zucchini sticks - 18 calories

1 cup cucumber slices - 13 calories

1/2 cup pickled vegetables (giardiniera) - 10 calories

2 tablespoons of salsa - 20 calories

Diet popsicle - 10 calories

1 dill pickle - 12 calories

Under 50 Calories

10 jelly beans - 40 calories

20 raisins - 35 calories

1 small peach - 35 calories

8 baby carrots - 32 calories

1 cup popcorn (air-popped) - 30 calories

1 cup tomato juice - 41 calories

1 cup strawberries - 43 calories

Nonfat cappuccino - 43 calories

Fast Food Facts

Eating on the road can play havoc with even the best laid dieting plans. Order grilled rather than fried, avoid fattening dressings, and go for small size servings.

Subway has a sandwich called the Veggie Delite. At just 237 calories and 3 grams of fat, it's a great way to eat on the run.

Kentucky Fried Chicken features Red Beans and Rice at just 126 calories and 4 grams of fat.

Dairy Queen's DQ Sandwich is just 140 calories and 4 grams of fat.

Burger King's Chunky Chicken Salad is only 142 calories and 4 grams of fat.

Arby's Roast Chicken Salad is 149 calories and 2 grams of fat.

McDonald's features Grilled Chicken Salad Deluxe. It's a great choice at just 120 calories and under 2 grams of fat.

McDonald's McGrilled Chicken Classic has 260 calories and just 4 grams of fat.

Wendy's sour cream and chive baked potato contains 80 calories and 6 grams of fat.

Eat Pasta

Pasta is a highly satisfying food that won't put weight on you as long as it's not swimming in sauce. It's easy to cook and store, and can be used in a variety of dishes. Since it contains mostly

Steam it Up

For added nutrition, steam your vegetables. Boiling destroys vitamins. Microwaving vegetables is also preferable to boiling them.

starch, it also slowly rations out energy. It's one of the slowest burning foods.

Eat Soup

Start a meal with soup or use it as a nutritious snack and you'll stave off hunger pangs. Tomato soup, made with water, contains just 85 calories a cup. Throw in some vegetables for vitamins, a few beans for fiber, and you've got a nutritious meal.

Make It Spicy

Not only do spices make low fat foods more desirable and satisfying, they also rev up the metabolism. Start a collection of dried and fresh herbs and spices.

Easy Substitutions

Instead of cream use evaporated skim milk or yogurt.

Applesauce holds moisture in. Use it when a recipe calls for oil or butter.

When a recipe calls for sugar, taking as much as 25 percent out will not affect taste.

Sprinkle powdered sugar over pancakes instead of syrup.

Spread your bagel with low fat jelly instead of cream cheese.

Use mustard instead of mayonnaise in your sandwiches.

Use wine vinegar instead of vinaigrette in your salad.

Top a baked potato with salsa in place of butter.

Frost a cake with marshmallow creme instead of frosting.

Suck on This!

A Tootsie Pop has only 60 calories, and its chewy center makes it more satisfying than a regular lollipop.

Drink Your Coffee

No matter how hard they try, scientists can't prove that coffee does any real harm. There are even recent studies that indicate that drinking fresh brewed coffee can up your antioxidant quotient.

Fill Up on Celery

Because it takes up so much space in your stomach, celery is the snack choice of the world's most beautiful bodies. It's a great source of fiber and a natural cure for constipation. It also contains both calcium and magnesium.

Choose Cereals for Fiber Content

Not all cereals are created equal. Choose cereals with at least 5 grams of fiber. Good choices include: Shredded Wheat, Grape-Nuts, Raisin Bran, and Granola. There are several others. Also be aware of calorie content. It varies greatly between cereals and brands.

The best thing about cereals is that some super-fortified varieties contain 100 percent of the Recommended Daily Allowance (RDA) for many vitamins and minerals. If you eat on the run, or skip meals, these cereals are an important source of nutrients.

"I eat my cereal as a snack, a quick dinner, and often carry sandwich bags of it in my car. I find it a filling, rewarding treat. It's fun to try the different varieties. It breaks up the monotony of getting in my fiber. I even treat myself to the occasional sugary children's cereals."

Mary, age 48, 33 pounds lost

Select the Right Cut of Meat

The fat content in meats varies from 1 percent for 4 ounces of skinless turkey breast to 9 percent for 4 ounces of beef sirloin. Allow for this when planning out your meals.

4 ounces of:

Skinless chicken breast has 4 grams of fat

Beef eye of the round has 5 grams of fat

Pork tenderloin has 7 grams of fat

Pork chop has 8 grams of fat

Lamb shank has 8 grams of fat

One pound of fat is 3,500 calories.

Good Eggs

A large egg has only 75 calories and 1.6 grams of fat. Use eggs as an inexpensive source of protein. After years of getting a bad rap, the poor egg is finally off the diet hit list. Plus, eggs are an important source of vitamin K, selenium, and riboflavin.

Foods for Good Looks

You wear what you eat, no doubt about it. Why not let your diet nourish your looks as well as your body?

Sweet Potatoes: Vitamin A is known to be a remarkable antiwrinkling agent. Sweet potatoes are full of this important vitamin. The pleasing result is clearer, smoother skin.

Wheat Germ: If you want to get rid of pimples quickly and efficiently, make sure to include two or three tablespoons a day in your diet. Add it to cereal, yogurt, and cottage cheese.

Cheese: To ensure a happy smile, add a slice or two of hard cheese into your diet. Choose Swiss, cheddar, or gouda to block bacteria in the mouth and prevent cavities.

Satisfy Your Cravings

Want to crunch? Choose pretzels or pita chips. Need something smooth and comforting? Low fat puddings or frozen fruit pops are ideal.

Don't Bother!

Although it's important to eliminate fat in our diets, don't worry about taking out whole milk from coffee. You only save about four calories, and many dieters believe that skim milk makes their coffee taste too watery.

All Lettuce Is Not Created Equal

Choose color when it comes to salad fixings. The darker the color, the more vitamins and minerals. Butter head, Romaine, and loose-leaf contain larger amounts of iron than the typical iceberg salad lettuce.

Dessert Ideas You'll Really Use!

Put whipped cream on top of sugar free Jell-O. It tastes sinful, and will add only 8 calories with a single gram of fat.

Combine orange marmalade with orange liqueur. Drizzle over orange slices. Dollop with whipped cream.

Core but don't peel an apple. Dust inside with cloves, cinnamon, and a little brown sugar. Bake for 30 minutes at 375 degrees.

Pop some popcorn and spray with a little nonfat butter spray. Sprinkle with cinnamon and a packet of sugar substitute.

Break Your Bread

Cut your pizza into little pieces and tear up your bread. The value of cutting your food into smaller portions lies in making your food last longer so you're satisfied with less. Dipping your bread into salad dressing, sour cream, and other condiments works the same way.

Prevent Bottom Feeding

Sitting down in certain places signals us that it's time to eat. Trigger areas include the couch in front of the TV, movie theaters, sporting events, or your mother's kitchen table. Even cars can be culprits. Get a motivational tape to play while you drive. Chew some gum while watching TV. Hold your honey's hand in the movie theater. Make alternate plans when you know your hunger will be triggered.

What to Eat Each Day?

You should choose foods that you enjoy, of course, but you need to include the following:

Vegetables:
Three to five servings. Try to include one serving of raw, leafy greens.

Meat:

Have no more than three 3 ounce servings a day. Cut off all fat. Try to make two servings of turkey or chicken. One serving of fish a day is ideal.

Fruits:

2 to 3 servings daily. One-half cup of chopped or sliced fruit is a serving.

Dairy:

At least two servings daily. A serving would be 8 ounces of milk or yogurt. 1¹/₂ ounces of cheese is a serving.

Fats

Salad dressing, cooking oil, butter, and mayonnaise should be limited to 2 servings a day.

How Big Is a Portion?

Trying to figure out what is the right amount to eat during a diet can become a challenge and an annoyance. Of course, you're not about to bring out the diet scale at the table in order to figure your portion size. However, your hand can tell you all you need to know. Your palm is the size of a 3 ounce portion of meat. Your fist is a cup, while your thumb is just about right for one ounce.

Stretch Out High Calorie Foods

Use low calorie fillers in dishes that pack a lot of calories. You'll still get the taste and satisfaction. For instance, add an extra portion of steamed rice to Chinese dishes. Double the lettuce and tomato in a sandwich. Add some sprouts to your potato salad.

"I look for fruits that have a high water content, and never eat any fruits that contain a lot of sugar. I'm trying to lose my sweet tooth. I'm also staying away from grapes because they are higher in calories and I tend to lose count."

Rachel, age 24, 14 pounds lost

"Whenever I eat fruit, I keep the pit in my mouth for about fifteen minutes. Sucking on the pit keeps the flavor in my mouth, and makes me think I'm still enjoying the fruit."

Genna, age 28, 26 pounds lost

"I need to fool myself a lot in order to stay on my diet. I grate almost everything I eat. This includes carrots, cabbage, and even apples. It gives me so much more volume. Sometimes I mix the carrots, cabbage, and apples together with a little vinegar and mayonnaise for an enormous cole slaw!"

Jinks, age 31, 20 pounds lost

"I love the taste of almonds. I use low calorie almond extract on fruits, cottage cheese, yogurt, even in water. It tastes absolutely sinful with no added calories. Flavor is everything to me."

Mona, age 61, 33 pounds lost

Chapter Five

Looking Good While Going Down

Dress Up for a New You

Don't wait until you've lost the weight to start to care about your appearance. Do it now, while you keep going down. You will not only look more attractive, but you'll feel so much better about yourself.

Rules of Dressing Thinner

1. Match your hose to your shoes. Legs look longer and thinner when hose is toned to skirts and shoes.

2. Pleated trousers conceal tummy bulges, so if this is your problem use those pleats to your advantage. The pleats must not be too full, though.

3. An A-line skirt can emphasize body length while hiding heavy thighs.

4. Use a shirt like a jacket or a tunic. Choose a generously cut shirt in a heavy or lined fabric. It's an elegant look over slim pants, flowing over every possible sin.

5. Dress in one color. Wearing one color from shoulder to shoe streamlines the body. It's called monochromatic dressing. If you don't want to limit yourself to just one color, choose colors that are closely matched. If you really want to go for "thin" stick to darker colors.

6. If you have a chubby neck, choose v-neck-lines. They create the illusion of a longer, leaner body.

7. To bring attention to the face, and away from the body, wear a choker and matching earrings.

8. A long jacket is a "pounds parer." It can make any outfit look elegant while hiding figure flaws.

9. Choose a low heeled shoe that is cut low on the instep. Stick to a thinner, more graceful heel.

10. A loosely fitted vest can hide a thick waist.

11. Wear belts in a low slung manner, or gently held around the waist.

12. Always wear control top pantyhose with Lycra.

13. A body suit can eliminate bulge. It also gets rid of unsightly "panty line" and fabric pulling.

14. Choose a well-fitted jacket. A look that is too loose or boxy tends to add pounds.

15. Simple styling is most slimming. Cuffs, pockets, and buttons can add width to the body.

16. Wear prints only at the slimmest part of your body. Stay with smaller prints, rather than big flowery ones. Florals have direction like any other print. Look for designs with vertical or diagonal movement.

17. Look for fabrics that drape the body. This would include light woolens, cotton, and rayon.

18. Stay away from very large shoulder pads. They may seem to add balance, but they're really only adding bulk.

19. Double breasted and breast pockets should be avoided if you're top heavy.

20. Lightweight knits can be slimming, if not worn too tight to the body. Let it skim the body, rather than cling to it.

21. Choose sturdy shoes, even heels. Delicate shoes make thick ankles look thicker.

22. A sarong skirt tied in front hides a tummy.

23. A shorter length makes for a leggier look.

24. A gently nipped-in waist trims the middle of the body.

25. Vertical buttons and seams lengthen the torso area.

Stand Tall! You'll look thinner, more confident, and more attractive with good posture.

Hair Styling Tricks

A good stylist can take pounds off your face with the right haircut.

Layers are the most important tool a stylist can use in slenderizing the face. Full cheeks become sculpted by creating angles starting at the temple and ending just below the cheekbones.

A **round face** can be lengthened by creating wispy bangs cut in an upside down "v" pattern. The shortest section of the bang will be at the center of the forehead.

Double chins can be easily camouflaged by beginning layering at the jawbone just below the ear lobe. Finish layering just below the chin.

Blow drying hair on a large round brush directly onto the face reduces width, frames your best features, and is extremely sexy.

An elegantly **upswept hairdo** with loosely gathered tendrils around the face brings attention away from the body.

Highlights create long vertical lines and the illusion of slimness.

Height in the crown of the head will instantly lengthen the face.

Consider **lightening** your hair by a shade or two. It will open up the face, and instantly slim down cheekbones.

> "The bigger the hair the smaller the hips."
>
> —Fran Drescher

Bronzing Powder—A Dieter's Best Friend

Looking to slim down your face with makeup? Head to your local drugstore and pick up an inexpensive bronzing powder. Use it to slim down your nose by running it down the sides. Create the illusion of cheekbones in a much more subtle and believable way by running the bronzer under the cheekbone area. Disguise a double chin by running the bronzer under the jaw line.

Can't find any bronzing powder? Choose face powder in a color two shades darker than your foundation.

Other Makeup Tips

Highlight Your Chin, Forehead, Nose Bridge, and Brow Bone

Dust a translucent face powder over the tip of your chin to emphasize its length. Use over the nose to focus the attention on the top of the nose, rather than the sides. Bring attention to the outside of the eyes by sweeping powder just below the outer portion of the eyebrow arch.

Play Up Your Brows

Bringing attention to your eyebrows will take focus away from that double chin, puffy cheeks, etc. The brow is known as the "frame for the face." Darken your brow a bit, eliminate any stray hairs, and be sure to brush upward. Keep your brows in place with a bit of hair spray. Spray it on an old toothbrush (or even on your index finger).

Emphasize Your Eyes

Line the lower rim of your lids with a white pencil. Curl upper lashes with an eyelash curler. Apply at least two coats of mascara to the upper lashes only. Apply shadow only at the outer corners of the eye in the shape of a sideways "v".

Elongate Your Hands

Little tricks you can use on your nails will benefit in your hands looking longer and thinner. Switch to a lighter shade of nail polish. Stay with beige and pink tones, so that they will blend right into your skin. If your nails are short, lengthen them by applying polish only on the center portion of the nail. Leave a sliver of bare nail on either side.

Fake a Good Body

Male and female models do it all the time. They work their muscles just before a photo shoot. If you have an event coming up, don't panic! You too can create a temporary "pumped" look. Here are some things that you can do just before going out so that you can really look good in that body revealing outfit.

1. Holding a ten pound weight, slowly lift it up and out to the side, bending arm at elbow. Slowly lower.

2. Holding a ten or twenty pound weight behind the head with both hands, slowly lower hands to the middle of the back. Be sure to hold elbows close to the head. Repeat 20 times.

3. You CAN wear that backless dress. Lift your arms straight out to the sides and squeeze shoulder blades toward each other. Count to ten and release. Do this at least 15 times. Holding 5 to 10 pound weights will yield optimum results.

4. Fake long sleek legs by raising up on tiptoes for as long as you can. Try to go a full minute. Raise up and down quickly. This will give your calves a firmer, more toned appearance.

5. Wear the highest heels you can walk in without killing yourself.

6. Hit the shower with a moisturizing body exfoliator to slough off dead skin on arms and elbows.

7. Shave with a moisturizing cream to avoid nicks.

8. Cover blemishes with a good concealer even on your shoulders and back.

9. Fake cleavage by dipping a brush into bronzing powder and dusting a half moon contour on

each breast. Start from above the breastbone, and go over and up to the armpit. Do this very subtly and no one will ever know.

10. Apply a self-tanner all over your body.

Beat the Bloat

Use these model's tips to look more svelte in even the most body revealing clothing.

1. Never drink from a straw, and never chew gum. Both will send air right to your tummy and distend and bloat you.

2. Avoid starches like pasta and bread. These foods cause the body to produce excess insulin, which puffs you out.

3. Eliminate salt for at least twelve hours before putting on anything body revealing.

4. Eat a few bites of protein. Turkey and fish are excellent choices for energy, and they'll keep you bright and wary of the fattening stuff.

5. Don't drink soda, not even diet. Doing so will give you a false, "fatter" body fat reading. The reason is, that it puffs up your body temporarily, even though there are no calories. It's the sodium that causes you to retain fluid responsible for this condition.

6. Rush blood to specific body areas for a more defined appearance.

A. Balancing on your knees, squatting on the floor, lift your arms to your ears and then lower to your sides in one controlled movement. Do 3 sets of 10 each.

B. Lie down with your legs raised in the air, knees slightly bent. Tuck your hands behind your head. Slowly lift your buttocks a few inches off the ground, squeezing them together as you lift. Hold to a count of 20. Lower slowly. Do this at least 25 times.

73

C. Hold onto the back of a chair, legs spread apart, and toes pointed out. Squat until your thighs are parallel with your feet. Do this 30 times.

Swim Wear

Primal fear

I have heard more primal screaming coming out of dressing rooms at swimsuit time than at any other time of the year. It doesn't matter what size you are or what age—does not matter at all! Trying on swim wear has to rate right along with the stirrups in those doctor's offices. I'm not saying that buying a swimsuit will ever be fun, fun, fun, but I can make it a little less painful for you. Here goes:

Rule #1: Go up a Size

This is not what most women want to hear, but because swimsuits are made of less fabric than other garments, they tend to run a bit smaller than regular street clothing. A size 12 suit will be very snug on a woman who wears a size 12 dress, but will be perfect on a woman who wears a size 10. If you insist on trying on your regular size, be certain that you can bend, stretch, sit, etc., without any discomfort or riding up.

Rule #2: Look at Tags

Thank the designer gods for finally listening to us. They have developed swim wear that actually gives off the illusion of having lost ten pounds. You'll see it in the tag-usually these suits are called "minimizers." Again, try them on, because you may find them quite confining. It's nice to be tucked in, but who want to feel that they're wearing a girdle on the beach?

Rule #3: Don't Be Afraid of Color

There is no reason to stick to black or navy if you're trying to give off the illusion of slimness. Although darker colors do slim the body, vibrant shades like purple, magenta, maroon, and green also serve this purpose. You can also use color to accentuate the positive, while hiding any negatives. For instance, if you want to show off a terrific bosom, choose a bright color in the bodice area with a darker bottom. Don't be afraid of lines in the fabric. Vertical lines can be especially flattering, as well as geometric shapes and polka dots. They cause people's eyes to never rest on a specific body area. Patterns keep the eye moving.

Get Rid of That Big Handbag

Nothing ruins the look of a streamlined body more than a big old cluttered handbag. Take all the junk out, and throw away any bag larger than 10 by 13 inches. This is especially important for large breasted women who look totally top heavy with an oversized purse.

75

You Can Wear Shorts

They just have to be the right style. Sorry, no "Daisy Dukes" for you if you're not in perfect shape. Drawstring shorts can make heavy thighs look slimmer, and reduce down any waist. Pleated shorts slim down a puffy tummy and offer a longer line. Cigarette and Capri shorts instantly make your legs look long and lean. Chubby knees look great in the new just below the knee pedal pusher styles. Walking shorts with a wide waistband actually raise your waist.

Help for Pear Shapes

Pear shaped bodies are heavier below the waist, just like the fruit. The way to balance this figure type is to pad on top.

1. Look for bosom-maximixing details like epaulets, breast pockets, and large buttons and embellishments.

2. Look for Empire styles.

3. Layer a shirt or sweater over a tee shirt or turtleneck.

Help for Apples

This body type (large torso and breasts with thin legs) needs help minimizing the bust line.

1. Make sure that the shirt is fitting without gapping. An oversized shirt will only cause you to look even bulkier.

2. Choose a long pendant to lengthen the torso.

3. A vee-neck will elongate and slim.

4. Choose a top that hits the hipbone. Stay away from tucked in styles.

Looking Leggy

Legginess is in the eye of the beholder. There are easy ways to fake the look even if legs are not your strong point.

1. Wear a front-slit skirt. If you can carry off a long length, it will be even more leg lengthening.

2. Match footwear, hose, and skirt.

3. Wear opaque hose with short skirts.

4. Wear some kind of heel, even with pants. Remember, the more casual the look, the thicker the heel. Flats squish you like a bug.

5. Always choose slim pants over flared or palazzo styling.

6. Wear long boots if you've got thick calves and ankles.

7. Choose a pencil skirt over a full dirndl type.

8. Never wear shiny or textured hose.

9. Stay away from straps.

10. Don't even think about socks, even with pants.

Large Sized Fashion Flubs

Pleated skirts

Fabric without substance

Large patterns

Accessories that are too dainty

Teeny tiny handbags

Clingy fabrics

Frilly silly clothing (stick with classics)

Use Body Shapers

The right lingerie can slim and tone you in all the right places. It gives your body a new look before you even begin losing the weight. While you're going down, it can keep loose skin streamlined instantly!

Some Choices:

Power slips

Uplift shapers

Slimming pantyhose

Tummy toning panties

Have It Tailored

As you head down the scale, you'll find your clothes sizes changing quickly. Some things in your closet might be worth saving if you can find a good tailor or seamstress. Consider the costs.

Pants hemmed: $20 to $25

Sleeves hemmed: $30 to $35

Skirts hemmed: $35 to $50

Shoulders taken in: $100 to $125

Waist taken in: $25 to $30

Tapering jacket, pants, or skirt: $35 and up

Maybe You Should Throw Those Big Clothes Away

If this is it, and you're definitely going to keep it off this time, consider giving away your large-sized clothing as soon as they become too big. Telling yourself that they may come in handy one day will become a self-fulfilling prophecy. Don't do that to yourself. They will become a huge albatross around your neck.

Buy Them a Little Too Small

Purchasing just one or two things that are a little bit too snug on you will be the perfect motivator to keep going on your weight loss plan. You can hardly wait to get into them! But don't go crazy. You don't know for certain just where you'll end up, and those too-tight outfits could become too loose in a matter of a month or two. Dieters have told me that they underestimated their ability to lose weight, and wasted far too much money on "in-between" clothing.

Dress to Express

As your body comes out of hiding, so does your personality. Let your clothes and accessories give the image that you want out there. What do you want to say to people? Make certain the image that is out there is one that people will respect and admire. So maybe you're not feeling terribly good about your body right now. There's no need to shout that message out to the world. Dress as if you are feeling proud of yourself, and before you know it, you will be. Just keep faking it until you're finally feeling it.

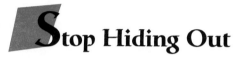

Stop Hiding Out

Put on the best outfit you can find, make it work for you, and just go out and start living in the world. Appreciate what your body has done for you so far in your life, adorn it with pride, and remember to honor it by treating it with respect and love with what you put on as well as in it.

79

Chapter Six

Secrets of Models and Celebrities

How Do They Stay So Thin?

Whenever anyone hears that I have been in the modeling profession for over 30 years and worked with the world's most glamorous celebrities, they always have questions. Surprisingly, the number one question I am asked is not "are they as nice or attractive in person?" Instead, everybody wants to know how models and superstars keep their bodies in such fabulous shape.

Are they born that way? No, not necessarily. What do they do? What's the big secret to their incredible shapes? The fact is that models and celebrities are just people. Yes, they are lovely looking people, but believe it or not, they have the very same problems that everyone has. Yes, they even have weight problems. The difference is their looks have become their fortune, so they have pulled every trick in the book to get thin and stay there. Their livelihood depends on it.

Ice Water

You've heard that models drink lots of water. Well, that's very true, but it's only half the story. To get optimum benefits from water, models drink ice water. With ice water, the body needs to use over 40 calories just to warm itself to room temperature in order to absorb the water into the system. That means that the theory of negative calories is true. You are actually using more calories than you are taking in.

Unfiltered Apple Cider Vinegar

What a versatile product! It's a great blood purifier when you put a tablespoon in a cup of hot water and drink it. You can also use it as an astringent for both your face and hair.

Colon Cleanser

No, I don't need to elaborate, but there is something to be said for the fact that if beauty is to really work, it needs to start from the "inside." Top actresses and great beauties throughout history have used this as an unconventional beauty/health regime. Legendary actress Mae West was famous for her daily enemas. Her skin was known to be as "soft as a baby's bottom" right up until the time of her death. These cleansers are now extremely popular, and readily available at health food stores in kits and capsules.

Kelp

Models carry kelp tablets to speed up their metabolism.

Dandelion Tea

This is used as a diuretic. Find this product in natural supermarkets and drugstores. Do stay near a rest room. Sometimes it works rather quickly.

Top Models Must Stay in Top Form

Cindy Crawford tends to gain weight in the buttocks area. That's one reason why she reportedly avoids dairy products. She has stayed at the top of her field because she treats her body as a direct reflection of her success.

Niki Taylor gained a self-admitted 70 pounds during her pregnancy, going from a size 6 to a 20. With self-determination and discipline, she lost it all, and was back on the runway after only 3 months. Niki is an avid runner, and is known to favor a mostly vegetable diet devoid of any dressings or sauces.

Jelly Beans

A jelly bean is a quick energy boost, and surprisingly low in calories and fat. Most of these little treats contain only 5 or 6 calories each. Compared with a LifeSaver (10 calories), or stick of gum (up to 20 calories), it's a pretty good way to snack. Models always keep these in their bags.

Eating just twice a day is a fact of life for many models, including **Elle Macpherson**. Each day it's a choice between lunch or dinner, depending on her schedule or mood. Those incredible abs of hers are a result of 500 daily sit-ups.

Her legs are the longest in the business, and her diet is varied, but disciplined. **Nadja Auermann** is the German beauty designers usually book first to show off their seasonal collections. She is a known vegetarian, and like so many in her league, uses beans in place of meats in order to get enough protein in her diet.

Claudia Schiffer is yet another model who eats lightly at dinner (salad and steamed vegetables), and eats nothing but fruits before noon. She is often seen on location snacking on tomato juice, black grapes, and herbal tea. While some of her fellow models prefer to engage in heavy exercise to stay in shape, Claudia prefers to stay slim with a stringent diet plan.

Her disdain for exercise has been a problem for model turned TV host **Daisy Fuentes**. In the past, her weight has fluctuated greatly and been noticed by critics. But giving up her favorites, pizza and hamburgers, and joining a health club, have been the answer to finally arriving at a lean, stable weight.

Few models have remained in the business longer that **Lauren Hutton**. No exercise fanatic, Lauren prefers taking long walks instead. She claims that water is her biggest secret to a youthful body. She drinks it all day, while basing her diet around salads, fruits, and vegetables. She rarely eats meats or desserts.

Few people know that **Linda Evangelista** is a great cook who makes delicious low fat dishes with creative substitutions. The only cravings she has are for meat, and she does allow herself an occasional hamburger. Since she is still actively modeling in her thirties, she is often seen at gyms pumping up her heart rate and toning her muscles on the treadmill and bicycle.

Beauty Has Never Been One Size Fits All

Audrey Hepburn was 5′7″ and weighed just 110 pounds. She was out of sync with the other screen stars of her time like curvy Marilyn Monroe, Jane Russell, and Jayne Mansfield.

A Childhood Weight Problem

Ellen star **Joely Fisher**, daughter of Connie Stevens and Eddie Fisher, was overweight growing up. Carrying an extra 35 pounds and the legacy of a drop dead gorgeous mom, Joely keeps her weight off by getting out in nature and hiking hills. She's come a long way since the days she was known as "Roly Poly Joely." Here's Joely's favorite method for getting 5 pounds off fast! Joely advises to stay on this diet for no longer than a week:

Breakfast: Low-fat yogurt and strawberries

Lunch & Dinner: Brown rice

Bulimia

Singer **Marie Osmond** has battled bulimia since she was a teenager. Although now living a healthy lifestyle, she confesses that she constantly battles the disease. She occasionally falls victim to a binge, eating an entire box of chocolates. She credits balance in her life, a supportive relationship with her husband Brian, and designing dolls (sold on QVC Shopping Network) for keeping her on track.

How Do They Stay So Slim?

Dateline anchor **Jane Pauley** munches on ginger snaps to get through her day without going off her diet.

Actress **Minnie Driver** relies on spirituality. She has been able to conquer a 30 pound weight gain and self-loathing to become one of the best success stories (and bodies) in Hollywood.

Ashley Judd maintains her 5´7˝, 125 pound figure with a heavy vegetable diet and by staying away from dairy foods. She begins her day with a drink of hot water and lemon, relies on herbs, and uses soy milk in her cereal. This southern belle grew up on fried chicken and biscuits, and still loves to bake.

Penelope Ann Miller makes sure she always fits exercise into her schedule, even when there's no gym available. While filming *Little City* she rode the elevator in her hotel to the 15th floor and walked to the 26th floor where she was staying. Rather than being carted to her trailer during breaks, she chose to walk (up to 20 times a day!). Adjusting her diet of skipping breakfast and eating a large dinner, she's changed her ways. Now she starts the day with a protein shake with nonfat milk and snacks on yogurt and fruit.

Demi Moore got into shape for *Striptease* by enlisting the advice of topless dancers. She used combinations of stomach crunches, walking lunges, and leg lifts. Demi keeps her system cleaned out by drinking herb teas and vitamins. "Having the tea between meals fills me up while the vitamins keep me going."

Baywatch babe **Gena Lee Nolin** lost her pregnancy weight by replacing starches with produce. She began eating mini-meals 5 or 6 times a day in order to keep up her energy and blood sugar level.

Curvaceous **Dolly Parton** eats everything she ate when heavy, but much smaller portions of it. She still enjoys her favorite snack of all, Velveeta Cheese, but just a few bites.

Jane Seymour satisfies her sweet tooth with frozen fruit bars. She had no problem getting her 5´4˝ figure back after delivering twins.

Former *Good Morning America* cohost **Joan Lunden** finds that eating low fat turkey breast helps her avoid sweets.

Fran Drescher is another "no dairy" success story. She has eliminated milk, cheese, butter, eggs, and ice cream to lose 28 pounds.

Singer/actress **Vanessa Williams** won't touch caffeine or wheat. How did she come to this dietary conclusion? She consulted a psychic!

Friends star **Jennifer Aniston** used to weigh 30 pounds more than her now svelte 112 pounds. This 5´5˝ cutie stopped eating mayonnaise sandwiches and fried foods and discovered the health benefits of low fat foods.

Suzanne Somers' weight problems caused her to lose acting roles. She credits a trial and error approach of combining certain foods in daily diet. She has also eliminated some foods that she labels "funky" that helped her get to lose 20 pounds. These include potatoes, white flour, sugars, caffeine, and alcohol.

Talk show host **Leeza Gibbons** uses "skinny" sauces like a combination of Dijon mustard combined with yogurt over baked potatoes. She eats dessert, but chooses fat-free angel food cake topped with fruit. Other snacks like popcorn, carrot sticks, and chocolate covered raisins keep at her weight of 130. This 5´8˝ beauty also hikes and runs, and uses the treadmill and stair stepper a couple times a week.

Actress **Melanie Griffith** is a busy mom, and can't always get to a health club. She keeps her 5´9˝, 118–20 pound figure by biking, swimming, walking, and running. She concentrates on eating right, and drinks bottled water and juices throughout the day. Melanie believes in supplementing her diet with vitamins and minerals. She changes them from time to time, depending on what her body is needing.

"Wonder Woman" **Lynda Carter** fits in exercise when she can, and absolutely insists that it be something enjoyable. Her favorites include skiing, hiking, running, and in-line skating. "That way it's not a chore," she says. Lynda stands 5´9˝ and keeps her weight at 130.

Turning 50 never looked better than it does on beautiful **Jaclyn Smith**. Her spectacular 5´7˝, 115 pound figure is the result of giving up cheese and cream sauces. She concentrates on meals that are low in fat, but still enjoys burgers. She is sure to include 45-minute power walks into her regime at least two or three times a week.

Who doesn't admire **Julia Roberts**' long streamlined body? Although she swears that she doesn't do anything "special" to maintain her 5´10˝, 120 pounds, during filming she is known for downing 8 glasses of water a day.

Cheryl Tiegs, Still Model Material After 50

How does Cheryl Tiegs, supermodel of the 60s and 70s, still maintain that fabulous body after passing that 50 year mark? Fitness is a constant in her life, and she stays on top of it on a daily basis. She claims to have kept a steady diet all her life.

Breakfast: it's something crunchy like Shredded Wheat or Grape-Nuts for fiber.
Lunch: the biggest meal of Cheryl's day, grilled meat, vegetables, and a salad
Dinner: fish, chicken, or meat with vegetables
Snacks: air-popped popcorn, occasional dessert

Exercise for Cheryl varies: aerobic conditioning, sit-ups, free weights, tennis, and hiking. The result? A weigh-in of 134 pounds every morning (she's 5´10˝). She watches her weight diligently.

Feeding Cravings

That's the secret behind Friends star

Courtney Cox. She is known for nibbling

on candy all day long on the set.

Admitting to a very strong sweet tooth,

Courtney compensates by eating lightly at

night. Running and power yoga also are

also a "must" in her daily activity to allow

her to indulge in her munching.

Secrets of the Soap Stars

Deidre Hall

This lovely star of *Days of Our Lives* tends to gain a few pounds if she's not careful. When she needs to lose weight quickly, Deidre uses a vegetable soup as a meal replacement. Although she loves Cheetos and dark chocolate nougat, her philosophy of eating is not to waste calories on non-spectacular foods. Her garden is tended by her two boys, and she encourages her family to eat fresh foods. Her favorite exercise? It's wrestling around with her boys, and jumping in the pool.

Susan Lucci

Don't hate her because she weighs under 100 pounds. Susan Lucci works very hard to stay so slim. She watches calories, and compensates for every indulgence. Although her favorite dish is pasta, she'll have it only at lunch so she can burn it off during the day. She carries her reputation for organization into her own kitchen, where she will often post weekly menus. Her favorite exercise is simply staying active.

A Big Problem Resolved!

Former Playboy Playmate of the Year **Anna Nicole Smith** blames her love of Southern-fried foods along with the death of her husband for ballooning her weight from 155 to 220 pounds. The 5´11˝ buxom beauty combined weight training and aerobic workouts to achieve her 60 pound weight loss to take off that gain.

Julia Louis-Dreyfus

The only woman brave enough to go up against the zany *Seinfeld* crew gained 65 pounds during her last pregnancy. Standing at a petite 5´3˝, she worked fervently to get back into shape. She limits red meats and concentrates on fish, pasta, fruit, and vegetables. Julia has worked with both a nutritionist and a personal trainer to resolve her post-pregnancy weight gains.

Listening to Her Body

It's hard to believe that gorgeous actress/comedienne **Lisa Kudrow** eats whatever she wants and yet stays a curvy 5´7˝ and 123 pounds. Her secret is listening to her body, and differentiating between cravings, physical hunger, and body satisfaction. Lisa claims that there is an inner voice that tells her when she's had enough to eat. Although there are no foods that she can't or won't eat, she limits herself to certain favorite sweets.

Relaxing about Food

Whenever former *Melrose Place* actress **Josie**

Bissett would eat a cookie, she would then figure out just how she could exercise it off. Stopping the obsession has given her peace of mind and greatly reduced her stress level.

Moderate Lifestyle Leads to Moderate Eating

The funny thing about model **Frederique** (best known for her layouts in *Victoria's Secret* catalogs) is that her diet is fairly normal. Born in the Netherlands, she was brought up in a culture where dieting is not part of the culture. She has brought with her the idea that it IS possible to eat one slice of cheese and an occasional piece of chocolate. Another crazy idea she's brought over from her country? She eats when she gets hungry.

How the Stars Handle Weight Gains

Actress **Salma Hayek** says that when she gains a few pounds she stops eating dinner for a few days. Her ideal weight is a remarkable 106 pounds.

Growing up in an Italian family gave **Mira Sorvino** a lifelong love of pasta, red wine, cannolis, and pizza. Mira has said that food is like sex: "When it's great it's amazing, and when it's OK it's still pretty good." When she needs to drop a few pounds, as she did to play a bulimic in *Beautiful Girls*, she sticks to salad, grilled chicken, and sushi.

Sharon Lawrence reportedly went on a crash diet to do her now famous nude scene in *NYPD Blue*. She survived on water and clear soup alone for several days before the shooting.

Being petite makes it even more difficult for **Toni Braxton** to keep those remarkable curves. Her figure has been the topic of great admiration. She loves to show off those curves with body revealing evening gowns. She got that way by practicing incredible restraint in the foods she selected. Hardest for her was eliminating beer and nuts (together they are deadly!).

A healthy lifestyle is the hallmark of longtime model **Christie Brinkley's** all-American body. This fish eating vegetarian keeps junk food out of the house to ensure that when weight gains occur, snacking is done on sweet potatoes and not candy bars. When she needs to lose weight quickly, she slims down on a liquid diet of fruits and vegetable juices, mixed with acidophilus.

When **Jamie Lee Curtis**, aka The Body, had to lose five pounds for her role in *True Lies*, she cut all fat from her diet and ate nothing but vegetables.

Kirstie Alley is subject to continual criticism of her weight fluctuations. Knowing that she has to stay competitive in the very visible acting world, she sometimes resorts to drinking only herbal teas for a couple of days.

Marilu Henner went from 160 pounds to 121 (she's 5´7˝) by eliminating all dairy products from her diet. She also eliminated all caffeine and refined sugars.

Statuesque *3rd Rock From the Sun* star **Kristen Johnsen** drops weight by cutting out desserts, between meal snacks, and butter on her bread. She substitutes lemon juice for salad dressing.

The Power of Protein
Although actress and former model **Cameron Diaz** has a fast metabolism, it may be her unusual way of starting her day that helps her keep her 5´9˝, 120

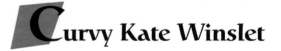

Curvy Kate Winslet

has been raked with public criticism ranging from fashion designers to show biz news groups on the Internet. Kate has battled her weight since her teenage years, and was called "Blubber" by her fellow classmates. She was able to diet down to a size six for her role in Titanic by eating sensibly rather than crash dieting.

93

pound perfect shape. Cameron eats a big serving of chicken! She claims it provides her with a quick energy start.

Actress **Lisa Rinna** chooses a chocolate protein shake for breakfast, blended with a banana. When she wants to drop a few pounds, Lisa cuts back on the amount of carbohydrates she's eating, and also adds more protein to her diet.

Figure skater **Peggy Fleming** stays low on carbohydrates and high on protein. Just a half cup of rice for dinner and a slice of toast for breakfast for this beautiful 50-year-old gold medalist.

Sensible Body Talk

Actress and former model **Andie McDowell** is a very healthy 5´8˝ and weighs in at 125 to 130 pounds. This proponent of a macrobiotic diet is a big opponent of the waif look of the model industry and the unhealthy lifestyle sometimes used to attain the image. You won't find her working out in a gym, but more likely riding horses on her family's ranch in Montana.

Revelations of Emotional Eating

Singer **Janet Jackson** explained in *Ebony* that food had become her favorite anesthetic. "I escaped through eating," she confesses. "Certain things may happen, and you dismiss them instead of stopping and saying, 'Why am I feeling this way? Why am I acting out in this way?'"

Defying Age

Sophia Loren is the doyen of discipline. For years she has talked about her love of pasta, but before you start digging in, listen to what she doesn't eat. Sophia rarely eats meat, and drinks lots of water. You won't find her eating potato chips, smoking cigarettes, or drinking an alcoholic beverage. Cheese, fruit, and vegetables make up the rest of her daily meals.

How does "Supreme" diva **Diana Ross** stay in shape? She does her own housework. "Cleaning is a tremendous stress reliever and it keeps my body taut," says Diana. Any 25-year-old would have a hard time competing with this 5´4˝, 100 pound 53-year-old.

"The body is a machine. You train it to do what you want it to do."

—Tina Turner

Yoga plays a major role in the wonderful condition **Raquel Welch** is in at 57. She practices some form of it every day. A big protein eater (turkey, veal, fish, some red meat), other snacks include rice cakes and fresh fruit.

Stirring honey into her coffee or tea helps **Ann-Margret** stay away from sweets. This motorcycle driving actress and singer watches her diet by avoiding soda, candy, and peanuts. She also reportedly went on a watermelon diet for two weeks to drop 20 pounds. She ate watermelon for breakfast and lunch along with lots of water. At dinner, she would eat a low fat, nourishing meal.

No snacks for former "Mamas and Papas" singer and *Knots Landing* actress **Michelle Phillips**. This 54-year-old owes her figure 5´7˝, 120 pound figure to fresh fruit and vegetables, supplemented by daily vitamins.

Faye Dunaway claims she is in better condition today at 56 than at any other time in her life. There is no white flour in her diet, just lots of salads, grilled fish, and vegetables, and seven-grain breads.

You can count **Goldie Hawn** as one of the lovely over 50 actresses who occasionally fasts on juice to detoxify and keep her in shape.

Barbara Eden of *I Dream of Jeannie* fame chooses lunch as her biggest meal of the day, because her body will have at least 10 hours to digest it.

Water and yoga have allowed **Ali McGraw** to remain 59 years young. She credits water with keeping her blood flowing, her muscles pumping, and her hair and skin healthy.

Catwoman **Eartha Kitt** likes to keep her weight at about 122. She's a mere 5´3˝, so if she finds herself five pounds over her ideal she increases her activity level by cleaning her house, and taking a two mile walk.

Dynasty's **Linda Evans**, now 55, has been able to lose 25 pounds thanks to 30 minutes of daily aerobics. She has so fervently embraced the exercise world that she has recently opened a chain of her own fitness centers. She is now able to keep her 5´8˝ frame at about 136 pounds.

Chapter Seven

Diet Emergencies

Crash Diets Can Work!

A crash diet isn't always a bad thing, and many times it really works! Emergency diets have the ability to inspire the dieter by the quick results seen over just a few days. Although the weight loss is mostly water, some fat is also lost. The other benefits are a flatter stomach, a sense of well being, and reduced bulges around the hips and thighs. Here are some of the most successful "quick start" diets.

The One Day Juice Fast

This diet is probably the most popular "one day only" diet (besides fasting) that has been used to drop about two to three pounds in one day without using any supplements. Fresh juices have great nutritional value, and contain important enzymes, minerals, and vitamins. They cleanse your system, and make you feel like you could conquer the world!

7 a.m.: A cup of hot water with the juice of one lemon or one teaspoon of reconstituted lemon juice.

8 a.m.: Apple-carrot juice consisting of 4 unpeeled carrots and two unpeeled, cored apples.

10 a.m.: A glass of water or a cup of herbal tea.

12 p.m.: A large glass of grapefruit juice and a large glass of ice water.

2 p.m.: A glass of water and a cup of herbal tea.

4 p.m.: A glass of pineapple juice and a glass of ice water.

6 p.m.: Herbal tea and a glass of water.

8 p.m.: Pineapple or grapefruit juice with a glass of ice water.

10 p.m.: A cup of hot water with the juice of one lemon or one teaspoon of reconstituted lemon.

If you find that you have a difficult time getting to sleep after a day of this juice diet, try adding a few special herbs to your bath. Visit your local health food store, where you'll find oils to help you relax.

Look for essences of rose, sandalwood, and lavender. To enjoy wonderfully natural aromatherapy, just cut up a lemon or orange and throw it in. These are the basis of citric cleaners, and will make your bathtub shine! Herbal tea bags also create a relaxing bath treatment. Especially soothing are cloves, peppermint, and chamomile.

The Cabbage Diet

This diet has been passed around forever. It's been called the Model's Diet, the Stewardess Diet, even the Dolly Parton Diet. I don't really know whose diet it is, but lots of people have had tremendous success with it.

Diet Soup Recipe
2 to 3 cubes of bouillon
1 package onion soup mix
3 onions

1 to 2 head of cabbage

2 to 3 pounds of tomatoes

1 carrot

1 pepper

Seasonings to taste

Blanche tomatoes in boiling water for one minute. Plunge into cold water, remove skins, and set aside. Dissolve soup mix and bouillon in 3 quarts of water. Chop and then add cabbage, onion, carrot, pepper, and spices. Add tomatoes. Bring to a boil and cook for 30 to 40 minutes. Makes enough soup for 2 days.

Eat all the Diet Soup you want for 7 days along with the following:

1st day: fruits only

2nd day: vegetables only

3rd day: fruits and vegetables

4th day: 8 bananas and nonfat milk

5th day: 6 ounces lean poultry or fish and plain rice

6th day: same as 5th day

7th day: vegetables and rice

"I've tried this diet along with everyone at my office, and it does work. The only problem is the weight comes off so fast that it's very easy to gain it back when you stop the diet. All my friends agree that it's a great way to get started on a new healthy lifestyle. On the day that calls for banana and milk, I make a milkshake. I also like to use a lot of spices on my fish, poultry, and vegetables."

Markie, age 27, 38 pounds lost

The Grapefruit Diet

This is a diet that doesn't require a lot of planning or thought. You don't need to count calories or make major food decisions. The plus side to this diet is that grapefruit contains so much fiber and water, it fills you up quickly. The downside is that it's too restrictive to be healthy for more than a couple of days.

Breakfast: Half a grapefruit with coffee or tea.
Lunch: Two eggs, lettuce and tomato salad spritzed with lemon and vinegar, a slice of toast, half a grapefruit, and coffee or tea.
Dinner: Fish or chicken, half a grapefruit, cucumbers or tomatoes, and coffee or tea.

The High Protein Diet

We saw the start of this craze with the late Dr. Stillman's Scarsdale Diet. It's still very much alive, and has been incorporated into many diets today. *The Zone*, *Protein Power*, and *Dr. Atkins' Diet Revolution* all are based on the protein theory that

too many carbohydrates prevent the body from burning fat. Typically the protein diet goes like this:

Breakfast: Eggs and bacon (unrestricted amounts), but no toast or juice allowed.
Lunch: Small salad and cheeseburger (no bun).
Dinner: Steak or fried chicken and a salad with blue-cheese dressing.

The Liquid Diet

This is certainly one of the most convenient diets around today. Slimfast, Nestle Sweet Success, etc., allow you to simply open a can, get a glass, and add milk. These shakes are nutritionally balanced and typically contain about 20 vitamins and minerals. The rule is to eliminate two meals a day with the shake, and eat a third meal consisting of no more than 500 to 600 calories. Each drink will contain about 200 calories and only 1 to 3 grams of fat. The problem that dieters face with this plan is that the oral satiety level is not fulfilled.

"I felt deprived on these 'milkshakes.' I was desperate to chew, and found myself sticking an average of 15 to 20 pieces of gum in my mouth daily. Although I initially lost a lot of weight, it gradually came back when I stopped using the shakes. I did like the convenience, and even now will bring one to the office in case I can't get out."

Penny, age 45, 22 pounds lost

The Mini Meal Diet

Eating food only three times a day, at breakfast, lunch, and dinner, is too restricting for many dieters. Being able to "graze" throughout the day, especially when cutting drastically back on calories, boosts the success rate radically. This plan allows for eating six times a day, and still will yield an average weight loss of five to six pounds in three days. It's easy to follow and really quite painless!

Menu One

Breakfast
1 cup Frosted Shredded Wheat with skim milk
Coffee or tea

Snack
1/2 cup cubed cantaloupe or one apple

Lunch
4 ounces sliced turkey breast on whole grain bread with 1 teaspoon mustard.
Mixed green salad
Coffee, tea, or diet soda

Snack
1 cup skim milk
1 chocolate chip cookie

Dinner

3 ounces broiled chicken or fish (any)

1 cup cooked spinach

Coffee, tea, or ice water

Snack

6 ounces low fat yogurt

Menu Two

Breakfast

1/2 cup strawberries

6 ounces low fat yogurt

Coffee or tea

Snack

1/2 cup baby carrots

6 pretzels

Lunch

1 cup canned vegetable soup

4 saltine crackers

Coffee, tea, or diet soda

Snack

1 apple

Dinner

3 ounces sirloin steak

1 cup sliced green beans

Coffee, tea, or iced water

Snack

1/2 cup low fat frozen yogurt

This diet works quickly and efficiently because you know that you'll be eating again in just two hours. Those of us who are parents know that when our children are young, it's important to bring along snacks if we plan to be away from home for a long period of time. Yet, we never anticipate our own hunger, which can lead to that stop at the vending machine, fast food drive-in, and the downfall of our best intentions of the morning. Snacking is important as an energy restorative as well as for staving off hunger pains.

Celebrity Crash Plans

Donna Karan

When designer Donna Karan wants to lose a few pounds quickly, she turns to her favorite detoxifying juice. In a food processor, blend the following ingredients: 1/4 wedge of cabbage, 1 red apple, 6 sprigs parsley, 3 carrots, 3 stalks celery.

Melanie Griffith

"I eat nothing but fruit in the mornings when I'm trying to lose weight."

Joan Collins

When actress Joan Collins needs to lose weight quickly in order to flatten her tummy into a slinky Dynasty type gown, she'll stop eating for an entire day. Sometimes all it takes is to eliminate one dinner.

Damage Control

Celebrities who make their living from the way they look immediately take care of any small weight gains. They don't let the problem run away from them. Their contracts, in fact their very fortunes, depend on it. It's a habit everyone should adopt into their lives.

General Emergency Measures

Stay Away from Sodium

Hide the salt shaker for a few days to shed those pounds quickly. Also stay away from canned soups, salty snacks, and processed foods.

Eat More Protein

Choose protein wisely and stay away from nuts and beans. Go for lean meats, poultry, fish, and egg whites.

Eat Less Carbohydrates

Limit your carbs to two a day and you'll find that the pounds will come off quickly. Your best choices are cereal (go for at least five grams of fiber), potatoes, and grain based breads.

Avoid Carbonated Beverages

Even low calorie drinks can give you a false bloated appearance.

Limit Added Fat

Try not to consume more than one tablespoon of salad dressing, butter, or other oil a day.

Eat Fat-Free Fruits

The fruits you select make a big difference in the weight loss game. Go for apples, pears, bananas, grapefruit, blueberries, and oranges.

Load Up on Fat-Free Vegetables

You can eat to your heart's content the following vegetables: green beans, broccoli, carrots, spinach, celery, mushrooms, tomatoes, and Romaine lettuce. Use these vegetables to refuel your body between meals, or whenever you get ravenous.

The Spa 3-Day Diet

Try this diet on a relaxing weekend. It's sure to bring a satisfying 5 to 6 pound weight loss. Try to incorporate it into a "makeover" time for you. Wear your workout clothes and take a hike around your neighborhood. Test out those homemade masks and hair treatments you've been anxious to try, but felt too busy.

Day One

Breakfast

2 frozen low fat waffles topped with 1/2 cup blueberries and a teaspoon of low fat topping
Coffee or tea

Lunch

1 cup mixed greens with 1 ounce water packed tuna and 2 tablespoons low fat dressing or mayonnaise

Drink Lots of Water

Don't worry, you are not going to add bloat by downing lots of water. On the contrary, the more you drink, the more easily your body will excrete it. When not enough water is absorbed into the body, a survival measure goes into gear, and the body holds on what it has. Don't forget to add lots of ice to rev up the metabolism. Water will also increase elimination.

105

Alfalfa sprouts and red peppers to taste

1 slice protein or whole grain bread

Diet beverage

Dinner

3 ounces chicken breast coated with 1 tablespoon each Dijon mustard, honey, and apple-cider vinegar Sprinkle with basil and broil

2 cups mixed greens topped with 2 tablespoons low fat dressing

Coffee or tea

Day Two

Breakfast

1/2 grapefruit

1 slice pita bread toasted with 1 ounce Swiss or muenster cheese

Coffee or tea

Lunch

Mix 1/4 cup grapes, pineapple slices, kiwi, and strawberries with 1 cup yogurt. Sprinkle with 2 teaspoons wheat germ.

Diet beverage, coffee, or tea

Dinner

1 cup pasta of choice topped with 1/2 cup marinara sauce and 1 teaspoon parmesan cheese

1 cup steamed zucchini

2 cups mixed greens tossed with 2 tablespoons low fat dressing

Coffee or tea

Day Three

Breakfast

1 slice raisin bread broiled with 1 tablespoons low fat cottage cheese topped with cinnamon

1/2 cup fruit

Coffee or tea

Lunch

1 slice pita bread broiled with 1 ounce mozzarella cheese, sliced tomatoes, and your choice of mushrooms, broccoli, and onions

2 cups mixed greens with 2 tablespoons low fat dressing

Diet beverage

Dinner

3 ounces white fish broiled with 1 teaspoon sesame oil and sesame seeds, topped with ginger

1/2 cup wild rice

1 cup broccoli

Coffee, tea, or diet beverage

Each day choose from two of the following snacks:

1 cup cubed cantaloupe

1/2 cup banana blended with 1/2 cup skim milk, 1 teaspoon vanilla, and 4 ice cubes

1/2 cup skim milk and 1 low fat cookie

Two Day Pasta Diet

Here's good news for pasta lovers. There's a fun diet going around that allows for your favorite food plus a 3 to 4 pound quick weight loss. Sound impossible? Try it, and you'll find it one of the easiest diets you've been on in a long time.

Day One

Breakfast

4 scrambled egg whites and 1/4 cup mushrooms

1 slice low calorie bread

Coffee or tea

Lunch

1 cup cold pasta mixed with 2 ounces tuna and 1 tablespoon low fat dressing
1 teaspoon grated cheese
Diet beverage

Dinner

1 1/2 cup spaghetti topped with 1/2 cup tomato sauce and 1 ounce browned meat
1 teaspoon grated cheese
Coffee, tea, or ice water

Day Two

Breakfast

1/2 cup low fat cottage cheese with 1/2 cup pineapple
1 slice low calorie bread
Coffee or tea

Lunch

1 cup egg noodles mixed with 1 ounce chopped chicken or turkey, 1 ounce melted part skim mozzarella cheese, and 1 cup cooked spinach
Diet beverage

Dinner

1 1/2 cups macaroni mixed with 2 ounces low fat melted cheddar cheese.
Mixed green salad with 1 tablespoon salad dressing blended with 1 tablespoon balsamic vinegar
Coffee, tea, or ice water

Chapter Eight

Supplements

Supplements for Weight Loss

You've heard it a million times. The safest and most effective way to lose weight is to eat less. If it were that easy, everyone would be losing all kinds of weight. Well, the good news is that there are supplements and herbs that really do work to provide that extra edge.

Chitosan

This natural fiber is found in lobster shells and acts like a fat magnet when taken 15 minutes before eating. Since it is nondigestible and binds with dietary fat, it quickly passes out of the body along with fat from the meal you've just eaten, report researchers. A study revealed that people taking Chitosan lost an average of eight percent of their body weight. The effect is reportedly enhanced when taken with orange or lemon juice before a meal.

Chromium Picolinate

Scientists have discovered that people who lack chromium in their bodies carry extra weight. The supplements chromium picolinate and chromium polynicotate have been around for a few years. Chromium is an essential dietary nutrient which plays an important role in processing fat and carbohydrates. Many users report that it cuts sweet cravings, too. You could use this supplement if your diet lacks in chromium rich foods. These foods include mushrooms, apples, broccoli, and cheese. The recommended daily allowance is anywhere from 50 to 200 micrograms. Supplements are usually sold in 200 micrograms, or mixed with other products in varying amounts. This product is readily available in drugstores, health food stores, supermarkets, and general merchandisers.

CLA

Conjugated Linoleic Acid (CLA) is a fatty acid marketed under the name Tonalin. Its purpose is to reduce fat by inhibiting the body's ability to store fats. CLA also increases muscle tone, improves food efficiency, and contains antioxidant properties.

Coenzyme Q10

Useful for obesity, coronary heart disease, lack of energy, and high cholesterol levels. Studies have found that some overweight people have low levels of Coenzyme Q10 (CoQ10) and by supplementing it they can help control their body weight. Recommended dose is for up to 90 milligrams of CoQ10 without side effects. Anyone with heart disease should first check with their doctor.

Creatine

This noncaloric enzyme can safely create better muscle tone and increase endurance for longer workouts. Creatine works by helping the body retain water in the muscle tissue, which helps to heal the muscle more efficiently without bloating the body. Recommended dosage is 10 to 20 grams a day for the first week, then 5 grams a day. Creatine monohydrate is available in capsules, bars, and shakes.

Garcinia Cambogia

Garcinia cambogia is a yellow fruit from Southeast Asia. Used in cooking, the garcinia extract is added to make meals more filling. Said to aid digestion, it contains hydroxyl citric aid, which is similar to the citric acid in citrus fruits.

Research conducted in the 1970s at Brandeis University, and later by Hoffman-LaRoche (the pharmaceutical company), showed that rats fed hydroxyl citrate shed 25 percent of their body fat in 22 days. The rats lost body fat partly because hydroxyl citric acid inhibits an enzyme that converts surplus carbohydrate calories into fat.

Available in pill form and in bars at health food stores, garcinia cambogia has taken the natural weight loss industry by storm. It controls the appetite in a natural, safe way, and has no known side effects. It is unlike any of the chemicals sold as diet pills.

Garcinia cambogia is a supplement that is most effective taken 30 to 60 minutes before meals. Take it with a glass of water or with a piece of fruit. Taking it with a bowl of soup also seems to help.

Glutamine

This amino acid promotes uptake of nutrients to build muscle tissue.

HMB

The latest fat burning and muscle building supplement to impress experts is beta-hydroxy-methylbutyrate (HMB). Studies showed that taking 3 grams of this protein substance daily caused athletes to gain 63 percent more muscle size and strength and lose twice as much fat as those exercisers who didn't take it

L-Carnitine

This supplement is reported to accelerate the benefits of chromium. Leading fitness buffs and diehard weight watchers take the two together. It is sold both as a separate unit, and in combination with other supplements. L-Carnitine is an amino acid which may be in short supply in many diets. The recommended dosage for this supplement is from 250 to 500 milligrams daily.

Meridia

This is a prescription drug that is meant to be safer than its predecessors, fen-phen and Redux. It will be prescribed only for people with a body mass index of 30 or above. Owing to the history of problems with other prescription weight loss products, it would be well advised to check that your physician has been properly informed about Meridia.

Orlistat

A new prescription diet drug that works directly on the intestine. It is part of a group of drugs called "lipase inhibitors." Lipase is an enzyme in the intestine that breaks down fat. This drug works on that enzyme to prevent the absorption of fat by about 30 percent.

Phen Cal-106

A combination of amino acids that works against the major causes of weight-gain, cravings, and binging. Originally developed to deal with substance abuse, the amino acids feed the brain. The brain becomes satisfied. You can also purchase the four amino acids in this product separately at your local health food store. They are: phenylalanine, glutamine, tyrosine, and tryptophan.

Pregnenolone

A hormone that is produced naturally in our bodies that decreases after the age of 35. Not only does it contain anti-aging benefits, but it makes it easier for people to lose weight and improve muscle. It also improves skin tone. Recommended dosage is 10 milligrams two or three times a week.

Pyruvate

Found in red apples, and now available in capsule form, this natural substance has almost 30 years of research to back up its claims and safety features. Use it to help burn fats and carbohydrates more efficiently.

Sibutramine

A new prescription-only appetite suppressant that works by maintaining high levels of serotonin, the blood chemical that triggers fullness. Those taking it experience fewer cravings and eat less. The most exciting results of extensive studies is that it enabled two out of three people to lose 5 to 10 percent of their body fat safely and without additional dieting or exercising.

113

Vanadyl Sulfate

This nutrient helps build lean muscle tissue by increasing amino acid uptake.

A Word about Appetite Suppressants

For those of you who use over-the-counter diet aids to suppress your appetite be aware of the following:

Purchase the cheapest brand available. They all contain the same basic ingredients.

Don't take more than the recommended dosage. There have been reports of strokes and deaths related to the misuse of these products. It is always recommended that you check with your doctor before taking them.

Herbs That Help Shed Pounds

There are herbs you can add to your diet as supplements, teas, and foods that will help your weight loss program go smoothly. Some can even be sprinkled into your bath.

Alfalfa

Aids digestion and acts as a diuretic. It belongs to the special vegetable family of nitrogen-fixing legumes.

Aloe Powder

Causes temporary water weight reduction because of its strong laxative effects.

Aloe Vera

Helps to maintain regularity, among its other benefits.

Bladder Wrack

Improves thyroid function and is a bulk laxative.

Burdock

Improves fat metabolism and acts as a diuretic.

Capsicum

This will produce heat to rev up the metabolism and burn fat.

Cardamom

Improves circulation and digestion. A thermogenic herb.

Ch'i-111

This all-natural herbal formulation (pronounced Chi-3) blends 12 herbs from China, India, and the Amazon rain forest with Western nutrients. Its purpose is to help create thermogenesis in the body. This will speed up the body's removal of fat from the adipose tissue (white fat). It also acts as an appetite suppressant. Follow the recommended dosage on the product's label.

Cayenne

Improves circulation and digestion. Has thermogenic effects.

Chickweed

Long reported as a weight loss tool by herbalists, but not widely tested scientifically.

Cinnamon

Creates a thermogenic burn.

Dandelion Root

Aids fat metabolism by affecting the liver.

Ephedra (Ma Huang)

Without a doubt the most controversial herb on the market today. Some have called it "legalized speed." It stimulates the nervous system, suppressing appetite. It also allegedly speeds metabolism. The side effects are dizziness, jitters, insomnia, and heart palpitations. Abusing the dosage has led to stroke, heart attack, and seizures.

Fennel

A diuretic that reduces hunger and improves energy.

Flax Seed

A bulk laxative that helps curb hunger. Flax swells in the stomach and intestines to promote a sense of fullness.

Garcinia Cambogia

Aids fat metabolism and reduces hunger.

Green Tea

Aids fat metabolism and increases energy.

Guarana

Helps to reduce hunger and has a laxative effect. It contains caffeine, and is reported to speed metabolism and burn fat.

Gymnema Tea

Is your problem a sweet tooth? Gymnema tea coats your tongue, tricking it into finding real sugar bland. The effect lasts for two to three hours. Dieters report that it takes away their desire for doughnuts, cakes, cookies, etc.

Hawthorn

Reduces blood fat and improves circulation.

Kava

This distant cousin to black pepper contains ingredients that produce physical and mental relaxation. Especially useful for stress related eating.

Kelp

This is a sea plant that is available in capsule form. It helps thyroid function, which regulates the metabolism.

Kola Nut

A stimulant that decreases appetite and aids in the metabolism of fat.

Papaya

Aids digestion.

Parsley

A diuretic and nutritional aid.

Phyllium

Helps to curb hunger and allow the elimination of wastes from the body.

Senna

An all-natural laxative. It is found in weight loss teas to stimulate the colon. To be used occasionally. Just like any other laxative, it can become habit forming.

Spirulina

Also known as blue-green algae, spirulina contains a natural appetite suppressant. It is a rich source of phenylalanine, a naturally occurring substance that helps create a feeling of fullness after eating.

Stevia

A little-known South American herb called Stevia rebaudiana-bertoni has not one calorie, yet is up to 300 times sweeter than sugar. Use it in its powder form to sweeten beverages. It's a natural alternative to aspartame and saccharin.

Valerian Root

If stress sends you right to the refrigerator, this natural tranquilizer will stop you from pigging out.

Vinegar

Ancient healers have used vinegar for thousands of years. Take two teaspoons of vinegar mixed with a glass of water at each meal. The vinegar will help your body to burn fat, rather than store it. Use any vinegar that appeals to you. Apple cider vinegar is a delicious flavor to try. Vinegar is a natural storehouse of vitamins and minerals. Experiment and come up with the tastes that you've never before experienced.

Aspirin for Weight Loss

An aspirin a day will burn away fat! The key is thermogenesis, the chemical process by which your body generates heat and speeds up your natural metabolism. Aspirin revs up the metabolism, making it run faster, burn hotter, and vaporize fat effortlessly. Less fat in the body can also unclog arteries and slash your risk of heart attack and stroke by 50 percent. Of course, you should check with your doctor.

Vitamins and Supplements for Health and Well Being

You are cutting down on calories, but you do not want to cut back on nutrients. In most weight loss programs, the requisite vitamins are not being consumed. Here are some of the supplements used to balance out a reduced calorie diet.

Bee Pollen

The buzz on bee pollen is that it gives you an extra

St. John's Wort

Known as the natural alternative to Prozac, it works to increase the production of the brain chemical serotonin, boosting mood and curbing overeating associated with depression. It's often used in combination with ephedra to battle weight problems, especially eating disorders and binge eating.

119

energy lift. Be sure to take small doses of it in the beginning. Some users have found that they are allergic to it. It's known as the "alternative to coffee" by holistic groups.

Cat's Claw

Known as the Peruvian wonder herb, cat's claw is the newest herb to come out of the ancient rain forest of the Amazon. A natural antioxidant, one of the major benefits is that it is anti-edemic (takes down swelling). Use it for swollen ankles, bloating, and PMS.

Dang Gui

Also known as dong quai and tang kuei, this is one of the most versatile herbs available today. From the name, it is obvious that its origins are in Chinese medicine. It has been used to treat menstrual abnormalities (cramps, PMS) and menopausal symptoms. It is also useful in treating respiratory problems, and even gas.

Echinacea

Rich in polysaccharides, echinacea helps to activate the immune cells. It naturally inhibits inflammation. Widely used in Europe, take it only when you feel an illness coming on. It has no cumulative effects.

Evening Primrose Oil

Particularly popular in England, it benefits the skin and hair, and is said to aid in hair restoration.

Folic Acid

Helps the immune system and blood building. Plays role in promoting DNA and RNA to make new cells.

Garlic

Take the deodorized tablets for benefits in lowering high blood pressure.

Ginger

It prevents motion sickness and relieves nausea. Ginger is also reported to prevent and heal ulcers.

Ginkgo Biloba

Good circulation is vital to supplying a healthy brain with the food and oxygen it needs. The ginkgo tree, derived from the oldest living tree, has many benefits. It increases alertness, improves memory, and lowers cholesterol levels. But more importantly (to our looks), there's evidence that ginkgo may be the most potent anti-ager ever! The only problem I have come across if that there's no agreed upon standard for the right amount to take. About 40 milligrams

Beta Carotene

This vitamin A precursor protects lipids in cell membranes and between skin cells from free radical attack. In everyday language, beta carotene makes the skin stay moist, supple, and youthful.

seems to be the recommended dosage from most sources I have solicited.

Ginseng

This popular supplement has many health and longevity benefits. It improves energy levels and enhances mental alertness. It has immune strengthening benefits and is able to lower cholesterol levels. Ginseng is reported to decrease the chance of heart disease and increase good cholesterol levels.

Grape Seeds

Antioxidants in grape seeds protect the thin walls of blood vessels from losing their strength. Beauties use it to prevent and correct the appearance of spider veins.

Grapefruit Seed Extract

Made from the seeds and pulp of grapefruits, grapefruit seed extract is receiving praise from both holistic and mainstream medical researchers. Its properties boost the immune system. It is also proclaimed to be an alternative to antibiotics. It is reported to fight bacteria, viruses, and parasites, which is why it is most used for flus, colds, sore throats, and even yeast infections.

Iron

A trace mineral that carries oxygen to cells to produce energy, iron helps the immune system operate at peak efficiency.

Kombucha Mushroom

This health craze is a living organism of bacteria and yeast, and has been used for centuries in China and Russia. One of its key ingredients is said to be glucuronic acid, a detoxifying agent. Devotees say kombucha tea improves well-being and energy levels. It's sold in many forms, and many beauties are making teas out of it, grow it—everything but wear it. I have heard some negatives about its safety, so do be careful. Some health professionals are concerned about the safety of the brew. If you would like to give it a try, I'd go with the tablet form, available at drugstores and vitamin outlets.

Lavender Oil

Use it in drop form in the bath, to alleviate stress, and to ease headache pain.

Licorice Root

Long used in Germany, this helps with vitamin absorption and the prevention of ulcers.

Melatonin

A supplement that in addition to being the ultimate sleeping pill, eliminates jet lag, and improves mood. It is also reported to enhance the immune system, treat a variety of diseases, and even prolong life. The biggest claims that have been reported (but as of yet unproven) are that it can reverse the aging process, fight cancers, and even prevent pregnancy. Most doctors, scientists, and nutritionists agree that from one to three milligrams is the recommended dosage.

Pycnogenol

A compound form of the French maritime pine, this is a most powerful antioxidant that acts in a similar way to vitamin E, but with fifty times the strength. It boasts twenty times the strength of vitamin C. Use it to protect cell membranes from sun damage.

Royal Jelly

This is one of the most enduringly popular food

supplements. Swathed in the mysteries of ancient China and the East where it was first discovered, royal jelly, in its raw state, is a unique high protein food. It is produced by bees and fed to their offspring. Used by us as a food supplement, it is available in both capsule and liquid forms. Loyal followers prefer the liquid because it can be more easily absorbed into the system. Also use it to boost your energy levels.

Seaweed

What you used to avoid at the beach has many health benefits. It's sold in both dried form and tablets. You can reconstitute it and add it to your salads and soups as many models do. If seaweed doesn't exactly tempt your taste buds, go for the tablets. The most popular tablets are Dulse and Kelp. Take it for the rehydrating benefits. Seaweed is also able to boost a sluggish thyroid.

Selenium

Take this vitamin to enhance the effects of vitamin E. Selenium has a close metabolic interrelationship with vitamin E, and will aid in body growth.

Vitamin A

Take this supplement to regulate skin hydration, aid eyesight, and repair skin and nails.

Vitamin B

This important vitamin keeps skin smooth, promotes hair and nail growth, and improves circulation.

Vitamin B-1 (Thiamine)

Stabilizes appetite, stimulates growth, and helps metabolism

Vitamin C

Available in several forms, it is quickly becoming the darling of the cosmetics industry. Vitamin C prolongs the life of vitamin E, protects immune cells in the skin to fight off cancer and other sun-related diseases. It also has been proven to fade age spots and other pigment irregularities. Of course, vitamin C also fends off colds.

Vitamin D

Promotes absorption of calcium and phosphorus and helps deposit these minerals in bones and teeth.

Vitamin E

Known as the skin vitamin, it has properties to heal scar tissue and neutralize damaging free radicals.

Wheat Grass Juice

Here's yet another purported natural energy enhancer. It is also used in homeopathic healing of some diseases.

Of course, you should try to get some of these nutrients in a multivitamin so that you're not spending half your day downing vitamins. That said, you'll become aware of what your body requires. Also note that vitamins should be taken with meals to help your body absorb them.

Chapter Nine

Exercise

Getting Started

You need to exercise. You'll lose weight faster and more efficiently if you do. Of course, exercise is also good for your health. The good news is that you don't need as much of it as the media has hyped. You simply need to start moving that body of yours. I'm sure you agree that we can easily become exhausted physically and mentally by some of the extremes celebrities and trainers go to on a daily basis to stay in shape. Who has the time, or for that matter who cares to spend two or three hours in a gym every day?

Exercising Doesn't Require a Bunch of "Stuff"

A lot of dieters fail to incorporate an exercise program into their dieting plans because they think they can't afford the pricey equipment. You can certainly get a good workout with lots of equipment or by joining a gym, but it's truly not necessary. The successful dieters I interviewed for this book didn't credit their stair stepper or treadmill with being their key to long-term accomplishment.

Exercise Can Boost Creativity and Imagination

According to the *British Journal of Sports Medicine*, men and women ages 19 to 59 scored better on creativity tests after a low or high impact workout. Studies also proved that mood was increased by 25 percent after exercise.

You Just Have to Move

Do something you enjoy for 30 minutes a day. Hey, it might just be gardening or housecleaning. Walking to the library to find that perfect book or video is a good motivator as well. If you combine these 30 minutes with a low calorie diet, the pounds will fall off, and that will become daily gratification.

Consult Your Doctor

Although your physician may very likely jump for joy when you mention it, it's a good idea to get checked out before beginning anything strenuous.

It Doesn't Matter the Time You Choose

According to several studies, including major research from Kansas State University, the number of calories burned will be roughly the same no matter when you work out. This was also the case with my own interviewees. The difference is that two-thirds of the calories burned by early morning exercise comes from fat deposits. It's cut to one-half if exercise is done in the afternoon or evening. Quite simply, though, the best time to exercise is when you're most likely to do it.

Make an Appointment with Yourself

This is your time just for you. If you can't find 30 minutes in your day, break it up into two 15 minute blocks. Imagine your body to be a piece of clay. You are the sculptor, and you know just how you want your arms, hips, and thighs to be sculpted. You'll be amazed at the strong, firm results.

Find a Friend

The right friend can make all the difference in the success of an exercise program. Is there someone who's commiserated with you on their own weight problem? Do you know anyone who tends to be naturally competitive? Perhaps there's someone in your family who's been after you to lose weight? Knowing you have someone else who's cheering you on, or even that one person you know you have to answer to, is the concept that makes most diet clubs so successful. Even better, if you can get that person to engage in that exercise with you, you are going to stick with it.

Maybe Your Mate

Working out with your partner may or may not improve your motivation and performance. It can bring you closer together if you stay aware of the sensitivities involved. It might be better to learn something new together than doing something only one of you is skilled at. Be sure to choose activities the both of you will enjoy. For instance, if one of you hates the cold, don't go skiing.

Turn Your Neighborhood into a Health Club

You won't pay any dues, and you won't be waiting in any lines by simply going out the door and walking your way into fitness. All you need is a well-designed athletic shoe. Make sure it comes with the proper cushioning. Choose clothing that allows for freedom of movement and remains comfortable in all kinds of weather. If you exercise at night, be sure to wear reflective fabric or attach reflective tape to ensure that you're visible to traffic.

Set Realistic Goals

It could be as simple as firing your housekeeper, and doing your own housework (that's what singer Diana Ross, Eartha Kitt, and others who can easily afford help do to work out). Perhaps it will be walking your dog more often, or just taking the stairs at work instead of riding the elevator.

You're Already Exercising

Almost everybody walks somewhere. The easiest way to start seeing results is to turn up the voltage on what you normally do. Add a weighted vest or hand weights if possible. You'll feel absolutely pumped!

The Proper Way to Walk

1. Pull your chin in so that your ears are over your shoulders.

2. Relax your shoulders.

3. Concentrate on pulling your tummy in tight and pulled in.

4. Walk with your arms bent at a 90-degree angle.

5. Tuck your elbows in close to your waist.

6. Try landing strongly on your heels with your toes slightly lifted for a more powerful push off.

7. Let your fingers relax.

8. Hold your wrists straight.

9. Breathe in deeply.

10. Your stride should feel controlled and smooth.

11. Keep your head up.

12. Your eyes should be straight ahead.

13. Be sure not to lean too far forward or back.

14. Let your arms swing naturally.

Walking for Health

Researchers have found that walking for an hour a day decreases the risk of colon cancer by half. Walking speeds digested foods through the body. As a result, toxins in foods spend less time in contact with the colon wall.

Take It to the Kitchen

Soup cans, soda bottles, and milk cartons make great weights. Use a sturdy kitchen step-stool to do buttock and thigh strengthening step ups.

Make Your Own Ab Machine

Get a bath towel and lie with it lengthwise under you. Hold an upper corner of the towel in each hand. The towel will support your head and neck while you do sit-ups and abdominal crunches.

If You Think You're Too Tired

Working out actually boosts your energy for long days, and helps you cope with stress. It also helps you sleep better. If you don't feel like exercising, tell yourself you'll just do 5 minutes instead of 30 minutes. Once you start, you'll probably want to keep going.

Get a Workout in Your Garden

If you hate sit-ups, the treadmill, and gyms, then get right to your garden. You can get the same benefits. Here's what to do:

Arms: heavy weeding and composting

Chest: digging and hoeing

Stomach: turning compost and raking

Legs: raking, hoeing, and digging

Back: raking and lawn mowing

Buttocks: weeding, digging, and mowing

Gardening just every other day will make a major difference in how you look and feel, and don't forget that gardening is known for giving spiritual nourishment. Spending just 30 minutes in the garden will burn off 150 calories.

Get a Jump Rope

Your childhood toy may just be the most effective piece of exercise equipment you could own. You've seen those incredibly fit boxers in training. You've seen them jumping away to shape and tone their arms and legs, as well as cutting fat. Jumping rope will burn fat, define muscles, and is one of the best cures for cellulite. Plus, it's fun, especially if you can remember some of your childhood jumping tunes.

"I like to bring a jump rope with me when I go for a power walk. I tie it around my waist, and since I walk where there are a lot of traffic lights, I jump while waiting to cross the street."

Sara, age 33, 28 pounds lost

Run if You Can

Even running short distances can yield great health benefits. Running just 15 minutes will burn 150 calories. Running up to 50 miles a week will yield high levels of HDL (good) cholesterol. Runners at this level also have half the rate of hypertension.

Dance Your Fat Away

Get your favorite tunes out and break a sweat! Tap dancing burns 400 calories an hour. The polka will take off 540 calories an hour. Swing dancing burns 300 calories an hour.

"My housework goes by a lot faster—and I exercise—when I put on my old school tunes. It seems like 'yesterday once more' when my stereo wails out those Beatles and Rolling Stones tunes."

Linda, age 47, 34 pounds lost

"I'm a very private person, but I love to dance. When everyone leaves the house, I become that disco diva and get my 30 minutes of exercise."

Ann, age 38, 40 pounds lost

Burn Fat without Trying

Brushing your teeth burns 140 calories a week.

Talking on the phone burns 2 calories a minute.

Playing cards burns 100 calories an hour.

Quality, Not Quantity

More is not always better, especially when you're doing an exercise incorrectly. Be sure to perform each movement slowly and in a controlled manner. Make sure you're in proper body form.

A Little Romance Takes Off

Dancing cheek-to-cheek for one hour burns 200 calories.

Machinery

Although no machine can miraculously give you tighter abs or lift that butt, you may be more motivated if you see it staring you in the face every time you walk into a room. If you're really interested in investing in a machine, you need to ask yourself the following questions:

How much should I spend?

Consider a second-hand piece of equipment if you can't afford a high-quality brand.

Will it fit?

One of the biggest problems is getting a piece of equipment home and discovering it won't go into the closet or even through the door.

"I set up my stair stepper with no problem. But when I went to use it, I found that my head kept hitting the ceiling. What a waste!"

Ben, age 46, 33 pounds lost

Will I really use it?

Even if you hate gyms, and the reason you're buying the equipment is to stay away from them, go for a few sessions. Get a guest pass if you can. See what machines you most enjoy. It might be too embarrassing to try out a piece of equipment in the store. Plus, you really won't get the entire picture if you just spend a minute or two using the demo model.

Stationary Cycles

Look for features like smooth pedaling and a comfortable seat. A stationary cycle is a good idea if cycling is your favorite workout and you want to keep up your routine during the cold winter months. Then when the weather breaks, you're in perfect cycling condition. There are many versions that fold down to a compact size.

Steppers

Look for higher hand grips, which make it a lot harder to "cheat" by leaning on the handrails. It should also allow you to climb at quick pace without sliding backwards. Look for pedals that move independently of each other. This will provide a

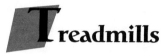

Treadmills

Before you plop down your money, be aware that this is the most boring piece of machinery you could buy. Think about it. You're going to run in the same spot every single day. However, a treadmill is a great option if you don't like to run in rain or snow, or if there's an unfriendly dog that has decided to move into the neighborhood.

135

more challenging workout. A wide stepping area is also desirable because it will be a lot more comfortable. Some of the steppers can be very noisy, so be careful if you enjoy listening to music while you work out.

Rowers

Look for steel or aluminum parts. They will provide longer wear. There is some maintenance involved, and a chain pulling system will mean less work. Toe straps should be very sturdy to be completely comfortable. Look for a rower that provides a smooth ride and a comfortable seat. Some of the models come with a race program, complete with an imaginary rower. Several models also include a back draft feature. All should feature distance and rowing pace, as well as a timer. Calories burned estimations sometimes are featured.

Strength Gyms

Look for floating bearings on all moving parts. This makes the machine superior to steel-on-steel construction. These machines should use aircraft-quality nylon-coated cable to connect the weight stacks to each station.

Cross Trainer

This machine is a cross between a bike and a treadmill. Look for resistance settings that can be changed. You might find this machine useful if you're recovering from a sports injury, or you can't take a lot of stress on your joints.

Machine Alternatives

It's not necessary to spend a lot on pricey equipment. You already have tools in your home that can make your workouts more effective.

Chairs

A simple straight-back chair can be used as an exercise tool. Here are three easy exercises:

To Firm Up Hamstrings

Stand straight and hold the back of the chair for balance.

With one leg, slowly lift your heel towards your buttocks. Hold for a count of five.

Return to starting position, then repeat with other leg.

Repeat ten times for each leg.

You should feel this in the back of your legs.

For Chest and Arms

Sit on the floor with your arms holding the chair's seat.

Extending legs in front of you, raise and lower yourself.

Thigh Trimmer

Sit on the edge of a sturdy chair. If possible, use ankle weights. Slowly straighten and lift one leg, then the other. While the leg is lifted, hold to a count of five. Repeat ten to fifteen times for each leg.

Exhale on the way up, and inhale on the way down.

Repeat ten times.

Books

A thick phone book or encyclopedia can work for several exercises, including popular "step" work.

To Shape Up Calves

Stand with your toes on a book, holding onto a wall or counter.

Slowly let your heels down as far as you can, feeling the stretch.

Rise again and hold to the count of five.

Repeat ten to fifteen times.

Scarves

Find a sturdy scarf that is at least a square yard in size for this exercise.

Tones Lower Back and Obliques

Stand straight, holding one end of the scarf in each hand.

Raise arms and pull scarf hard.

Twist the body as far to the right, and as far to the left as you can.

Do this ten to fifteen times.

Vegetable Cans

Vegetable and soup cans make perfect small weights for these toning exercises.

Pecs Enhancer

Create great cleavage by toning your pectoral muscles.

Hold a vegetable can in each hand. Lift your arms straight out to the side, with elbows slightly bent.

Bring your arms to the front of your body until the cans touch.

Repeat fifteen times.

No More Flabby Arms

Taking a vegetable can in one hand, lean over a chair and place your other hand on the seat.

Fully extend the arm holding the vegetable can and reach backwards and up.

Do this twenty times with each arm.

You'll know you should be doing this exercise if you arm still waves "good-bye" after you stop.

The Wall

Use the wall as a resistance tool.

"Kiss the Wall"

Stand about three feet from a wall, back straight, legs bent slightly at the knee.

Extend your arms straight in front of you, and rest your palms against the wall.

Bending your arms, lower your body toward the wall and "kiss" it.

Push yourself back and repeat twenty times.

Bottle Beauties

1. Stand with your knees slightly bent, and grip a two-liter bottle. Keeping elbows close to the side, move lower arm up and down. Repeat ten times with each arm.

2. For great shoulders lift bottles in front of you. Keep elbows and knees slightly bent. Move bottle to your eye level. Repeat twenty times.

3. Hold bottles at sides and bend knees and elbows. Slowly raise arms out to the sides up to the ears. Repeat twenty times.

Broomstick

A great tool for balance and lifting

Stationary Lunge

Holding onto the top of the broomstick, step back
with left foot.

Bend knees and drop hips until left shin is parallel
to the floor.

Both knees should be at right angles.

Rise from lunge position, lifting knee to a 90-
degree angle.

Alternate legs and repeat fifteen times.

Hey! Great Shoulders!

Developing your upper back will make you look
like you've lost five pounds!

No More Excuses

Time

Think of the time you waste each day. It may be on
the phone, flicking through TV channels, or brows-
ing the shops. You can always find time when it's
important to you. Even if you have to set your
alarm 30 minutes earlier, make the time.

Injury

Of course, certain physical conditions prevent
exercising. Most problems, however, can be
worked around. A physical therapist can set up a
program that's safe and effective for you.

Video Hype

With so many exercise videos on the market today,
how do you tell what's going to work without

wasting a lot of money? Here's a few things to look for:

1. Inspect the claims and don't fall for the "pie in the sky" promises.

2. Look for credentials. Check out certification, and don't fall for vague titles like "America's best fitness trainer."

3. Find the copyright date. New data on training pops up every day. Don't buy anything that's more than two years old.

4. See what else you might need. You might bring home a tape and find out that it's to be used with an ab roller and you don't own or want one.

5. Don't fall for lingo. If the box is not easy to understand, you won't be able to follow along with the video.

Chapter Ten

Special Problems

It Takes More Than Willpower

Even the best intended dieter will find certain glitches that make reaching their goals more difficult. This chapter includes those very problems that were mentioned consistently among the dieters I interviewed, along with the solutions they found.

The Four O'Clock Hour

The period that wrecks havoc with a well-planned day of dieting for many people is between 4 and 5 p.m. This is when all control is lost. Why? You probably ate your lunch at noon, and four hours later your stomach is empty. Your blood-sugar level is low, and your brain, as well as every cell in your body is saying "feed me." You're tired and vulnerable. Your first instinct is to grab something sweet. Although a sweet treat may quickly give you an energy burst, it will quickly fade.

"When I come home from work, I take a nap. I've finally figured out that I'm not really hungry, and can last until supper. This is thirty minutes that I use to restore my energy without food. It gives me the energy to gain control of myself so I don't 'pig out' at dinner, and can get some exercise after eating."

Pam, age 45, 20 pounds lost

"I eat a small salad with a glass of ice water. It helps me to eat less at dinner."

Pete, age 30, 22 pounds lost

"An apple and a cup of tea hold my appetite until dinner."

Cindy, age 35, 25 pounds lost

Low Fat Foods

The problem with eating only low fat or no fat foods is that dieters tend to eat more than they should. This is because foods that are lower in fat are generally less filling. Sometimes they'll end up eating more of the low fat food (calorie-wise) than they would if they just ate the regular version.

"When I would use low fat dressing on my salads I would pour on double the amount. Now I use my regular salad dressing, and extend the flavor by mixing it with a little vinegar. My salads taste better, and I don't have that chemical taste I find with low fat dressing."

Linda, age 27, 30 pounds lost

"I don't feel so deprived when I eat regular foods. I've just learned to count out the number of chips I eat, the amount of ice cream, etc., and I'm much more satisfied, and able to stay with my program."

Chuck, age 51, 45 pounds lost

Friends and Family

It could be your mother, your best friend, or your significant other. Those closest to us sometimes become our diet's worst enemies.

"My mother's house is like an eating orgy. I tell her that although her food was delicious, if I eat another bite, I'll get a bad stomachache. She's still a mom, so my health is more important to her than my enjoyment of her cooking."

Mary, age 29, 20 pounds lost

"My husband traditionally brought me chocolates for Mother's Day, Valentine's Day, my birthday, etc. So now I just tell him ahead what I really want. If he plans to take me to a restaurant, I always ask to choose the location, and then call ahead to make sure they have low calorie choices on the menu."

Cindy, age 36, 32 pounds lost

Boredom

A sure way to get tired of staying on a diet is to eat the same foods each and every day just because they're "safe" foods, or because you won't overeat

Cravings

The problem with cravings—and you're going to have them—is eating around them. For instance, you're dying for a cookie, and you end up eating three cups of popcorn instead. What you should do is just eat the cookie in a small portion, and your craving will be fulfilled without major problems. Afterwards, if you're still hungry, you may find there was really something else going on with that craving.

that particular food. Then you become bored out of your mind and go back to your favorite foods, the ones that got you into trouble in the first place.

"Once a week, I try out a restaurant with a different cuisine. It might be Thai, Portuguese, or just a brand new place in town. I concentrate on vegetable-based dishes, made without a lot of sauce. I've never gained weight, and it satisfies my senses. Plus, it just makes my diet more fun."

Jenny, age 48, 25 pounds lost

"I've started collecting cookbooks. There are great cookbooks out there that have the calorie and fat content listed right along with the recipe."

Mary, age 29, 20 pounds lost

"Every couple of weeks I visit ethnic and 'whole health' supermarkets. My taste buds have completely changed. I'm eating foods I never dreamed I would grow to love. Not only do these new foods make me feel adventurous, but a lot healthier!"

Sharon, age 33, 27 pounds lost

Stress

Feeling stressed out leads to craving the comfort foods of our childhoods. It really is possible to keep these foods in our diets. I know many models who look forward to that cookie at the end of the photo shoot. The difference is that they don't devour the whole bag, and the emotional satisfaction is still there.

New studies show that chronic stress not only creates added weight, but also creates hormones that can contribute to "abdominal obesity," strongly linked to diabetes, heart disease, and stroke.

Prolonged stress creates increased levels of "steroid hormones" which act together with insulin, the pancreatic hormone triggered by eating.

Skipping Breakfast

Many dieters fail to eat breakfast, the most important meal of the day, because of time constraints or because they think they're saving calories.

Reasons to Eat Breakfast

1. You'll have a better day at work. Dieters who eat breakfast work faster and more accurately than those who don't. Breakfast eaters are also more creative in the morning.

2. It keeps you in shape. Breakfast eaters are slimmer than those who skip breakfast. They don't reach for doughnuts or croissants at the first coffee break.

3. You'll have lots of health benefits. Cereal with skimmed milk and fruit will boost your vitamin intake for under 200 calories.

Unsatisfying Foods

If you're hungry all the time, there's no way you'll stick with any diet. But there are food choices that will provide more satisfaction than others, and they aren't the foods that you think. The best choices include:

Popcorn

Oatmeal

Legumes

Fruit

Baked potato

Look for foods that are high in water content, fiber, and protein.

147

Fat Thinking

"Fat thinking" is such a problem that there are gorgeous creatures walking around with the mentalities of fat individuals. They pay attention to every pound, putting them on an emotional roller coaster. They get depressed by the scale, and then they eat because of their depression.

"I don't weigh myself more than once a month (I used to do it twice a day). The way my clothes fit and how I feel is a more accurate guide."

Alexis, age 25, 30 pounds lost

"I've learned to accept a compliment. I used to think someone saying something nice was the result of kindness. Now I try to absorb the compliment as truly mine."

Rachel, age 40, 53 pounds lost

False Hunger

Real hunger means that you physically need to eat. It is usually accompanied by a gnawing, almost hurtful feeling in the pit of your tummy. Just wanting to eat is very different. It is most likely a direct reaction to an external cue (TV ad, power of suggestion, a smell, etc.). We might even eat because someone near us is eating. Identifying the triggers that lead to eating when we're not hungry is the first step to overcoming it.

Are You Sure It's Hunger?

There are physical signs that will let you know if you're just experiencing a craving or if you're really hungry.

1. Headache, a light-headed feeling, or irritability.

2. A need for anything carbohydrate.

3. Increased salivation.

4. Stomach noises.

"When I'm in a restaurant, all I have to do is look at a pastry cart, and I'm 'gone.' What has helped me is to order a specialty coffee ahead of the dessert menu, and to ask the waitress not to bring the cart by."

Susan, age 38, 40 pounds lost

"I've given my kids an allotted cookie allowance. They even have a strong box where they lock up their treats, away from me. It's taught them the value of money, as well as the value of rationing their snacks."

Alecia, age 32, 40 pounds lost

"The midmorning coffee break was a time when I mindlessly ate without thinking about it. It was only when a gorgeous coworker joined the group

Brush Your Teeth

That awful taste you have in your mouth when restricting calorie intake can lead to eating. Instead, brush your teeth and tongue with a flavored toothpaste.

and sipped coffee without the requisite jelly doughnut that I stopped and thought about what I was doing. Of course, I was jealous out of mind over her great figure."

Cindy, age 41, 18 pounds lost

"Changing my route after work to avoid passing the bakery was the best thing I ever did for my diet. Now I pass by a yogurt shop."

Sam, age 33, 62 pounds lost

Do Something Else

Take a bath or go to a movie. Take a walk or call a friend. Do anything that will keep you busy until that hungry feeling goes away. Don't worry, eventually those cravings will subside.

Eat Bread

Sometime a single slice of bread can calm nerves and end that craving like no other food can.

Rest

It may be that you just need to relax for a few minutes. Don't try to restore your energy level with food.

If you're eating less, be careful when driving. A USDA study found that drivers on a low calorie diet have a slower reaction time.

Get Your Protein

A small protein-rich snack can eliminate that craving by keeping blood sugar and energy levels balanced.

Watch Out for Allergies

Researchers have discovered that constantly craving a particular food may mean that there is an allergy lurking in the ingredients. Ask your doctor to test to see if you might be allergic to wheat or dairy.

Bloat

Bloating is a problem that has many reasons, but is truly bothersome and uncomfortable. Avoid foods that are rich in fat, alcohol, cabbage, artichokes, and carbonated drinks. Beer is one of the key sources of bloating. A few strategies for reducing bloating are:

Increase fiber intake
The colon will relax, and this will help aid regularity.

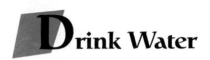

Drink Water

Add a lot of lemons to take away

that awful empty feeling that

cravings bring.

Exercise

Even just walking after a meal will allow gravity to take its course.

Eat regular meals

Strict diets reduce the traveling time of food throughout the gastrointestinal tract which results in bloating. Make breakfast your largest meal, and make certain dinner is not too large or too rich.

Cut down on spices

Too many spicy foods can irritate the gastro intestinal lining.

But Don't Bother With:

Laxatives

Your intestines will become dependent on them.

Colonic irrigation

Research indicates that it can alter bacterial flora which normally aids digestion.

Snacking

Eating between meals is not the problem. It's what you choose that hurts.

"The only way I can get through the day when I'm dieting is with a few snacks. That's why I keep a calculator and ration my snacks (my choice) to 500 calories. I'd much rather have a smaller meal, and save the calories for my snacking."

Michelle, age 21, 20 pounds lost

"I schedule my snacks so that I can have one between each of my three meals. In the morning around 10 a.m., I have an apple and a bag of pretzels, at 2 p.m. I have a frozen yogurt, and at 4 p.m. I have a shrimp cocktail. The total in calories? Just 300."

David, age 43, 35 pounds lost

Winter Weight Gains

Many people put on the pounds during the colder months and it's not only the holidays that are to blame. People gravitate towards higher fat foods like casseroles, breads, and puddings in the winter months. They're much less likely to eat lower calorie salads, fruits, and fresh vegetables. Some of this may be due to the colder weather, boredom from being inside, etc. Some of it may come from depression caused by decreased light. You might want to consider a special light that is sold to combat "seasonal-affective disorder." Otherwise, choose whole grains and healthy vegetable-based soups for sweet or starchy filler foods.

"I used to let myself go in the winter, and then hide the weight under big sweaters and lots of layers. Then in the summer I'm shocked by what my body has become. I was sick of this yearly event, so I now keep my bathing suit in my bathroom and try it on every week. This works better than my scale at keeping me from gaining."

Marsha, age 40, 22 pounds lost

Fast Foods

Since most fast food meals are 50 percent fat (according to the *New England Journal of Medicine*), it's no wonder that the pounds can pile on.

"When I know that I'm going to be eating at a fast food restaurant, I cut back on my other meals to compensate."

Sandra, age 22, 16 pounds lost

153

"I look for healthy choices on the menu when my kids want to go to the nearest fast food restaurant. Usually they're side dishes (like salads), so I get two of them to add up to a meal."

Monica, age 31, 35 pounds lost

Binging

Everybody overeats from time to time. Continual binges can lead to major health and weight problems. If you do find yourself eating out of control, put your food down and yell "stop." There is a reverie associated with binging that can practically render you semiconscious.

"When I find myself overeating, I run into the bathroom and brush my teeth. The toothpaste breaks the hold the food has on my taste buds."

Donna, age 50, 20 pounds lost

Quitting Smoking

There is truth to the legend that smokers gain weight when they quit. A smoker burns more calories than a nonsmoker because the consumption of nicotine uses energy. Extra pounds gained when quitting can be avoided if you:

1. Drink water to flush the toxins out of your body.

2. Snack on raw vegetables to satisfy the oral anxieties suppressed by smoking.

3. Avoid caffeine-based beverages which may increase your appetite.

4. Try sucking on sugar-free lollipops if you need something in your mouth.

Sugar Addictions

If you constantly crave candy, cookies, chocolate, or anything else with a lot of sugar in it, it is a real problem. Try substituting sweet fruits like raisins or apples. Chocolate syrup used in moderation can give you that chocolate fix, and diet hot cocoa/chocolate is a very tasty product.

"When I feel the need for a doughnut or other pastry, I spread a little 'all fruit' jelly on a rice cake."

Pam, age 34, 100 pounds lost

"My treat of the day is a teaspoon of Cool Whip on a graham cracker."

Sid, age 50, 65 pounds lost

"A piece of licorice takes a long time to chew, and puts that sweet attack on the back shelf."

Cindy, age 25, 30 pounds lost

Airplane Food

Requesting a special meal when traveling takes just moments and can save an average of 500 calories. When you make your reservations, ask for a vegetarian or low fat meal. You'll get an entree that includes fruit instead of cake or a cookie, fresh vegetables instead of chips or crackers, etc. Special meals are also the first meals served to passengers.

155

"I freeze Hershey's kisses and suck on them like LifeSavers. They have become my true diet savers."

Susan, age 31, 140 pounds lost

Sagging Skin

The fear of every aging dieter is that they will look older by dieting because their face will sag. It is possible to lose weight and keep firmness in the skin. That's why nutrition is so important, and crash dieting should be avoided. Make certain to include plenty of protein in your diet to maintain firmness. Your body will repair itself with protein, but the lack of it will cause a lack of clarity and elasticity. Try to get in at least 100 grams of fish, eggs, cheese, and milk. It will make a major difference in your looks.

Other tips:

Drink less alcohol and always drink a glass of water as a chaser if you do drink.

Take a vitamin E and selenium.

Apply vitamin E to the skin. Break open a vitamin E capsule and add it to your regular moisturizer. It will protect your skin from ultraviolet light as well as reduce the appearance of fine lines and wrinkling. They sell antioxidant creams at the cosmetic counter for big bucks. It's not necessary to spend that money. A drugstore moisturizer, even Crisco, provides moisturizing benefits.

Late Night Munchies

If you are really hungry at night, you need to take a look at your dinner menu. Make sure that your dinner does not contain too many carbohydrates.

Although they will give you energy, they will only stay in your stomach for about three hours (about the time it takes for those munchies to creep up). Adding more protein will keep you feeling fuller for a longer time period (about six hours).

A glass of warm milk contains relaxing amino acids.

"This ritual has stopped me from eating before bedtime. I take a luxurious bath, complete with scented candle, new age music, and aromatherapy bath salts."

Kathy, age 46, 28 pounds lost

Constipation

A side effect of some diets is irregularity. Although the number one cure is adding lots of fiber, sometimes this is not possible. Here are a few other hints:

Drink lots of water (add lemon to flavor).

Drinking coffee (even decaffeinated) has a mild laxative effect.

Eat fruits, rather than fruit juices (especially apples and prunes).

Add a teaspoon of powdered vitamin C to fruit juice.

Menstrual Blues

Women gain, on the average, 4 to 5 pounds just before their period. It's an interplay of hormones that doctors tell me is just too complex to be easily explained, but there are ways to avoid this increase, such as:

Increase carbohydrates to keep your blood sugar levels up.

To prevent water retention, include bananas, spinach, and broccoli in your diet.

Take magnesium supplements.

Cut down on sodium and processed foods, including diet soda.

"I'm a girl. I have hormones. My body changes."
Courtney Cox explaining away her "fat" days

Setbacks

It can be a vacation, a weekend of partying, or a major life crisis. All setbacks and lapses prove is that we're human. It's not fatal. Here's how to get back on track.

1. Take immediate action. The sooner you start, the easier it will be. Don't try to analyze it to death.

2. Make it a priority. For the next few days, monitor everything you eat, and become proactive in your plan. After getting back on track, you can go back to coasting.

3. Create a schedule that will not leave you much time for anything else. Write down your menu, take a class, or get your hair done. Get back to you.

4. Don't do anything drastic. Don't try to fast or go crazy with exercise. It's a form of self-punishment which just won't work.

5. Avoid temptations. Throw away that party food and liquor, and decline that invitation that may lead to further problems.

6. Don't wear the bulkiest item you own. This just reinforces the negative feelings you have towards yourself.

7. Forgive yourself and get on with other important issues in your life not involving food.

Junk Food Junkie

What is this love affair with anything that comes out of a package? It's probably the convenience factor. You grab and go! What could be easier? Dieters I spoke with said that the appeal was usually based on impulse.

"With my job, I just don't have time to eat anything but prepackaged foods. I now carry around my food, but instead of a bag of chips, it's a bag of baby carrots. In place of a candy bar, it's a granola bar. It's still just as convenient."

Marty, age 25, 30 pounds lost

"Single portions help me regulate my eating. I pay a little more, but I can look at the package and see just how many calories I'm consuming, and I don't have to try to measure what I'm eating."

Cathy, age 38, 70 pounds lost

"I hate to cook, really hate it, and love to sit and eat out of a bag. There are some amazing choices out there I've found that contain nutrients and take no time to prepare."

Fred, age 48, 50 pounds lost

Family Chef

You take care of your family by cooking what they love. The problem is that you end up tasting and testing the very foods you've been trying to avoid.

"I have to spend a lot of time in the kitchen. The smells are intoxicating, and the only way I can stop myself from eating what I'm cooking is to keep a cup of bouillon at my side."

Tina, age 35, 48 pounds lost

"If I make my family a meal, I try to include at least two dishes that I can eat too. Then I can make one meal, not feel deprived, and get my family used to eating low fat foods."

Cassie, age 45, 69 pounds lost

"I'm learning to cook more simply by broiling meats, cooking without a lot of oils, and serving sauces on the side. My family doesn't seem to mind, and I'm spending less time in the kitchen where I'm always tempted."

Sue, age 27, 19 pounds lost

Expense

You can eat healthily and still lose weight on a budget. Some of the most nutritious foods are the cheapest, like rice, pasta, beans, lentils, frozen fish, and canned tuna. Avoid waste by cooking large quantities and then freezing meals in individual portions. Make your own sauces instead of buying expensive ready-made varieties. Make your own salad dressings, or thin down the bottled varieties. Fruit and vegetables bought in season are usually cheaper than the packaged variety.

"When I'm preparing a casserole or stew, I cut down on the meat and double up on the vegetable ingredients."

Chandra, age 26, 14 pounds lost

"I've found that some of the cheaper cuts of meat are also tastier. They just take a little bit more preparation. Some of the most expensive cuts I've bought seem to have the most fat. My family seems to like anything that comes off the outdoor grill anyway."

Frank, age 45, 53 pounds lost

"I've really started to eat more healthfully since I started growing vegetables in my own garden."

Paul, age 47, 33 pounds lost

High Cholesterol

There are naturally cholesterol lowering foods that will also lower your weight. Apples, beans, carrots, chili peppers, eggplant, garlic, grapefruit, skim milk, oat bran, onions, seafood, spinach, soybeans, and yogurt should be in your weight loss program anyway. If you have a high cholesterol count, make sure that you have plenty of these foods.

Aging

It's a very hard fact of life's process that as we age the pounds want to come on and stay on. This is unfortunately due to a more sedentary lifestyle that creeps in, as well as the natural process of aging. It does get harder to fight the fat as we get older, but it's not inevitable. Start eating less fat and exercising more. What we took for granted when we were young just cannot happen without the extra effort.

Plateaus

Having trouble losing those last few pounds is a very common problem. It's usually because dieters get tired of working so hard and don't stick as strictly to their diet as they have been. They start adding a few little treats that start to build up. Here are some tips for pushing past that plateau:

Do I Really Know What I'm Eating?

Spend three days writing down every mouthful, every pat of butter, and every taste treat you grab from a bag. Work out the daily calorie intake. If you're trying to lose those last few pounds, the total calorie intake should probably not be more than 1200 calories.

Do I Really Need to Lose Those Last Few Pounds?

If you're at a healthy weight, you may not need to lose more. Your body might be telling you "enough is enough." Take a look at your goal, and make sure that it's realistic and not some model image, or a weight that you think might look good on you.

Is This the Right Diet?

Choosing your own eating plan will be far more successful if you're almost there. Your willpower has been used and reused, and now you need to

make up a diet that works with the foods you love to eat. You've learned the principles of weight loss by now, so just apply them to those last few pounds.

"I wasn't losing that last ten pounds to reach my goal, so I cut back on cheese and red meat and started walking ten extra minutes a day. It made the difference."

Linda, 50, 40 pounds lost

The Refrigerator

Constantly going into that refrigerator can tempt you as much as entering the most delectable ice cream shop or bakery. You need to either clean it out or cover it up.

"My frig looks like a mass of aluminum foil. I can't stand looking at leftovers without salivating, so in place of plastic wrap, I've stored everything in foil with the proper labeling."

Mac, age 35, 58 pounds lost

"I put the bad things in the back of the refrigerator, and the low calorie foods in the front. Rather than digging through, I'll reach for whatever's handy."

Pat, age 34, 40 pounds lost

"It may sound silly, but I went to one of those joke shops, and bought one of those sound alarms. Whenever I open my refrigerator, it tells me to 'get out.'"

Meg, age 44, 17 pounds lost

"I put a picture of me, at my slimmest, in a bathing suit on my refrigerator. I leave the frig alone so I don't ruin the picture."

Sandy, age 30, 25 pounds lost

Chapter Eleven

Intimacy and Weight

It's All about Self-Perception

Both men and women relate weight with not feeling sexual or seductive. Women especially blame themselves for not fitting into society's so-called physical ideal of seductiveness. Yet most people do not and cannot fit into the ideal of the fashion magazines and screen (TV and movies) images. There is no data available to indicate that size has any effect on seductiveness.

So You're Not a Supermodel

Not many people are, but everyone's trying to look like one. Sex is not about how you look, it's about how you feel.

A Happy Love Life Can Help

Don't use the excuse that you don't have a perfect body to avoid sex. Sex can help you look and feel better. Just think of it as one of the more pleasant ways to lose weight.

Sex Is Good Exercise

Believe it or not, an amorous lovemaking session will burn off 500 calories in an hour. Hey, that's about as much as 40 minutes on a treadmill!

Sex Lowers Cholesterol

Scientists have found that your body's cholesterol level drops after a lovemaking session.

Sex Regulates Menstruation

If you are a victim of irregular menstrual cycles, check your sex life. Researchers have found that women who have sex every week are more likely to have regular menstrual cycles of 28 or 29 days.

Better Skin Tone

People who have sex regularly find that their skin tone is better, due to the level of hormones being raised. It may be the reason people who are in love look so radiant. These increased levels of hormones are also known to cause hair to grow faster and give it extra shine.

No More Headache Excuses

Throw away the aspirin. Hormones released during sex, such as progesterone, act as a mild anesthetic, easing pain and headaches.

Sex Can Make You Smarter

During sex the oxygen level in the blood is raised. This has an energizing effect on the muscles, and revs up mental ability.

Surprising Scents That Put You in the Mood

Pumpkin pie
Licorice
Doughnuts (mostly men)

Hygiene Is Most Important

Both men and women mentioned body odor as being their number one sexual turn off. No matter what your size, it has the most lasting negative impression. It is especially important to shower daily if you are very far from your final weight goal.

Fake It

No, I'm not getting that personal, and I don't mean to suggest you fake anything involved with the sex act itself. What I mean is that you should act like you are a godsend to the opposite sex and soon you'll begin to really feel that way. If you find yourself unattractive, so will everyone else.

"Even though I was a size fourteen, I was ashamed that I was not a size four. I rarely dated, and when I did, my dates never failed to comment on my

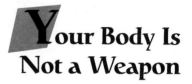

Your Body Is Not a Weapon

Don't use it as one against your partner. Some dieters I talked to told me that they actually gained weight in order to create a buffer. They put on the pounds because they knew that their partner would be upset about it. The result is that the dieter became even more unhappy.

weight. My best friend, who was two sizes bigger than I was at the time, not only had more dates than me, but also had a couple of marriage proposals. Unlike me, she was totally happy being a size eighteen. She had been a woman of size all her life, and walked into a room like she owned it. Even when I finally got down to a size eight, I still couldn't attract the type of guy I wanted. It was only through therapy that I was able to figure out that it had little to do with weight."

Rachel, age 40, 53 pounds lost

Don't Squeeze

Wearing clothing that is too tight is constricting and bothersome. You will feel more sexually confident with flowing clothes that feel good on your body. It will change the way you feel, and even the way you walk. Practice walking in front of the mirror the way models do. Put one foot in front of the

other, toes and balls of your feet before your heels, head held high. Tuck your tummy in and pull your shoulders back. This will make you look pounds thinner, taller, and you'll look and feel sexier. Walking a little faster will also get people to notice you.

Work Out Together

Grunting and sweating together is sexy! If you aren't physically up to a big workout, just taking a walk together will help you connect.

"My girlfriend and I are pretty competitive. When we started working out together it became our favorite foreplay."

Ken, age 27, 25 pounds lost

"I took my husband for a surprise hike on a very secluded path. We took some breaks."

Alexis, age 25, 30 pounds lost

Discover Self-Love

Look in the mirror, smile, and just say "hi!" That's you in there. Self-acceptance is harder when there's no feedback coming from outside sources. The more desperate we become for compliments and reaffirmation, the harder it will be to lose the weight. Concentrate on something you see in the mirror that you like, rather than your short-comings. If you have great hair, an engaging smile, or shapely legs, you have a tool that is significant to your self-esteem as well as to your sensuality.

"When I went from 125 to 185 pounds, I lost total confidence in myself. I felt completely useless and nonsexual. I pushed my husband away, in every way, even though he never sent me any negative vibes. I became reclusive, combative, and we eventually divorced."

Susan, age 32, 50 pounds lost

Celery, The Great Seducer

Men who have been practicing their best lines for seduction should shut up and start chewing. Scientists have found that the potent male hormone androsterone is found in celery. Androsterone is released through perspiration after eating. Although the smell of celery itself is undetectable, the hormone has the power to attract women. Side benefits include a high fiber, low calorie snack that freshens breath.

Coffee, The No-Calorie Turn On

Studies indicate that our morning cup of coffee may not only be getting us going, but turning us on. Men and women who have at least one cup of coffee a day are nearly twice as likely to describe themselves as sexually active. Men who drink coffee reportedly have less problems with erections.

Create Flattering Lighting

Certain lighting can bring flattering reflection to the skin tone. Photographers know this, and you can use it if you're less than confident about your body. Replace your lighting with pink- or blue-tinted light bulbs in your bedroom. A 20-watt incandescent bulb will do wonders! If you can't find any of these bulbs in your hardware or drugstore, just light a few candles.

Foods for Passion

There are foods that not only will help you lose those extra pounds, but will get you in the mood.

Apples
Remember what happened to Adam and Eve?

Bananas
Known as the fruit of love, the banana is revered in Asia and Africa. They are rich in potassium and B6, associated with female sex hormones.

Cinnamon
Known throughout the ages as an important romantic enhancement.

Dill
Use it as a tea, add it to breads or salads, or just eat a pickle.

Eggs
Folklore claims that eggs can cure sexual diseases. Today we know that they're rich in an essential amino acid that influences sexual arousal.

Figs
Rich in niacin and magnesium.

Ginseng
Very popular today, it was known in China to keep men virile. Take it as a capsule, drink it as a tea, or visit a Chinese supermarket for other foods.

Green Tea
Said to strengthen body fluids.

Honey Pollen
Stimulates the reproductive system. Add it to yogurt or cottage cheese.

Lavender
It can be added to sauces and desserts.

Lemons
Supposedly adds staying power.

Mussels
It could be just a visual, but it's been a constant. Plus it's rich in iron.

Mushrooms
They are great by themselves, added to antipasto, broiled, or marinated.

Nutmeg
A little goes a long way as a sugar substitute.

Oysters
Rich in zinc, they are undoubtedly the favorite aphrodisiac—and with good reason.

Parsley
It also gives you fresh breath for kissing! Almost NO calories here.

Peaches
The fruit of passion for their suggestive shape and soft touch. A great source of vitamin A, which manufactures sex hormones.

Raspberries
Another vitamin A source.

Scallops
Makes for sensual eating, and is very low in calories.

171

Sunflower Seeds

A good source of phosphorus directly impacting sexual desire.

Wine

Just a little as a spritzer. Too much is too many calories and will put you to sleep.

Chapter Twelve

Children and Weight

The Growing Weight Problem in Children

In the United States at least one child in five is overweight. In Australia the number is one in four. The number of overweight children continues to grow. It increases yearly, and has doubled in just the last two decades. The chances that an overweight child will suffer lifelong weight problems are high, and dieters who have been overweight at a young age find losing the weight in adulthood is that much harder.

How It Happens

Although genetic factors play a major role in childhood weight, there are also environmental components. The two top reasons listed by overweight adults were a lack of physical activity and unhealthy eating patterns. The most severe cases of childhood obesity recollected a combination of the two, whereas adults who described themselves as "chubby kids" listed only one of the above.

What Is Overweight in a Child?

A doctor is the best source for determining whether a child has a weight problem. A pediatric physician will not only look at the requisite height, weight, and frame criteria, but will also consider age and growth patterns. In rare cases, doctors have found an endocrine disorder that is evaluated through blood tests.

"I thought that my 12-year-old daughter had developed a weight situation that I wanted to address, since I had battled my own weight for many years. Her doctor told me that her body was in the normal range, and she had entered a 'prepubescent' phase that was age appropriate. Although I monitored her eating patterns, it did subside in about two years."

Polly, age 45, 68 pounds lost

Lifestyle

The amount of activity in a day plays an important role in a child's weight. Too much television, computer time, and video games are the biggest contributors to a sedentary lifestyle in children. The average child spends a full 25 hours each week watching television. Turning over just half of this time to sports or other physical activity would make a monumental difference. Another reason behind childhood obesity is that so many children are home alone after school and can snack on whatever they want, and as often as they want.

Children and Body Obsession

Recent studies indicate that children as young as 6 or 7 already may be concerned about their image, and become afraid of gaining weight. The desire to be thin can lead to children starting to diet in the primary grades. Although parents should do their best to set forth a positive body image in their children, unconsciously they may be sending out signals that contribute to a child's obsession with body image. It is imperative that both parents develop their own healthy habits, because children will learn by your example. Family activities should center around exercise and movement. It is important that parents develop children's socialization skills, building both their self-confidence and self-esteem.

Diets and Kids

Putting a child on a diet can lead to interference with the normal growth cycle. Physicians rarely put children on restrictive diets. Instead they work with the parents to develop a positive eating relationship with their children. Conversations at mealtime will slow down the speed of eating. This gives the stomach's fullness signals a chance to

Family Dynamics

Children whose parents or siblings have ongoing weight problems are at greater risk of being overweight themselves. Although genetic factors can play a major role in increasing weight profiles, it is more likely shared family behaviors (eating, activities, social habits) that are the most influential.

175

work. Even small amounts of food will start sending satiety signals to the brain after about twenty minutes.

Schools Are Part of the Problem

Most school lunches have a fat content of about 45 percent. Although many schools are working to change to more healthy menus, educators cannot start too early with proper food choices. Also, be sure your child is learning proper nutrition in their classes, and that they are able to understand the types and relationships of different foods. For example, some schools are now teaching the five food groups by color.

"My son was about 40 pounds overweight at nine years old. He felt isolated, was picked last at sports, and had few friends. I was a total loss at what to do. I am a single mom, and his father lived out of state. I decided to put him in an after school care program at the 'Y'. They had only one snack period, and the rest of the three hours concentrated on all kinds of activities, not only sports. At first he absolutely hated it, hated me for sending him, and was combative with the program leaders. After three weeks, he started to enjoy himself and lost all his weight. Now he plays in three sports at the junior high school level, and is very happy. I feel that if I had not done something at the age of nine, I would have had a depressed child and major problems."

Tammy, age 41, 13 pounds lost

How to Help Your Child

1. Become a role model. Don't act like it's a sacrifice to eat low fat foods.

2. Don't keep unhealthy treats in the home.

3. Don't make separate meals for the overweight child. It will only make the child feel isolated.

4. Never use food to punish or reward a child. Giving a child a sweet as a reward will lead a child to believe that it has more value than other foods.

5. Discourage meals while watching TV, as well as snacking while doing homework. Have designated eating areas in the home.

6. Don't be too restrictive with foods. Don't label foods, count it, or otherwise put that kind of fear or control in your child.

7. Recommend but don't dictate. Offer a variety of healthy choices, and help your child to develop his or her own sense of taste.

8. Eat meals as a family whenever possible. Dine out when you can afford it. Teach your child that food can be fun.

9. Limit time in front of the TV, computer, and other sedentary activities.

10. Involve your child in preparing meals, including shopping.

Chapter Thirteen

Holidays, Vacations, and Other Trip-Ups

You Can Handle Those Special Occasions

There's no need to turn down an invitation, cancel a trip, or avoid an important family celebration because of fear of gaining weight. Just because you've made the decision to lose weight doesn't mean you have to deprive yourself of life's pleasures. You can't push life away while you diet. Even if you're at your healthy weight, you have to learn to handle yourself in the everyday circumstances of life. However, even the most disciplined dieter can become completely overwhelmed by the events and situations that take us from our everyday routine. Temptations, family pressure, and just plain inconvenience can undermine willpower and discipline. Here's how winners in the weight loss game overcame these difficult situations.

Thanksgiving

The very word brings to mind tender, fall-off-the bone turkey, glazed ham, pies, cakes, etc.—a proverbial eating orgy. More than any other day of the year, Thanksgiving is the one that begs to be forgiven for overexcess and sheer gluttony. Our rationalization of our overindulgence is that it's okay because it's only that one day, and we have all year to exercise and diet it off. Don't kid yourself. That one day can start off an eating extravaganza that will last the entire holiday season, and into the new year. The table at Thanksgiving represents abundance and its traditional dishes bring back fond family memories. Calories rule.

Turkey

White meat is lower in fat than dark meat. Five ounces of sliced, skinless white meat contains 219 calories. Five ounces of sliced, skinless dark meat has 262 calories. Also, substituting turkey drippings with a gravy base made from chicken broth will cut calories in half.

"I substitute maple syrup for butter to glaze the turkey. Then I baste it with some of the turkey drippings. It's delicious!"

Sally, age 44, 50 pounds lost

Mashed Potatoes

"We love mashed potatoes, but the calories are killer! I made a few changes to lower them by blending skim milk instead of whole and adding garlic to season. My family loved it, and I saved ten grams of fat from the original recipe."

Mary, age 48, 33 pounds lost

Stuffing

"Rather than the traditional stuffing baked inside the turkey itself, I make a cornbread stuffing that I moisten with broth. It doesn't taste greasy, and yet it's not too dry."

Pat, age 34, 40 pounds lost

Christmas

There's no reason to dread Christmas. It should be a favorite time of the year. There's enough stress with shopping, housecleaning, and scheduling time and people. Healthy living means moderation, not deprivation. Keep the traditions and foods of the season you've come to love by making some minor modifications. Be sure to remember the true spirit of the day. Family, friendship, and love are what this holiday means. It's not about pies, cakes, and cookies. Concentrate on the true spirit. Food is important, of course, but it's not what you truly want to remember about this holiday.

Make an Allowance

Save your fat calories if you've been dreaming about your sister's quiche. Eat lightly at other meals, concentrating on fruits and vegetables.

"If I know that I'm going to a big holiday party, I prepare myself by eating salads for dinner all week, and passing on too many snacks. Not only do I have the calorie allotment for that 'special' meal, but I look better in my holiday outfit."

Ann, age 38, 40 pounds lost

Be a Good Guest

Offer to bring a dish, and make it a delicious recipe that's also low in calories. You'll be a hero for helping out a busy host, and you'll have something you know that you can eat without trepidation.

"When I go to a party, I try to prepare myself before I go. I look over the table, and if I don't see anything I can eat, I just grab a beverage and get into the conversation. If I think I'm being watched, I put a couple of things on my plate and kind of move it around."

Dina, age 39, 25 pounds lost

When It's Your Party

Although you have the control here, you want to serve food that will really be enjoyed by your guests. If you only put out a bunch of celery sticks and carrots, it's going to make for some quick exits. Create a combination of choices so everyone there will find something to enjoy. That said, you can substitute skim milk for whole, egg beaters for whole eggs, etc., and your guests won't even notice.

Don't Eat the Decorations

It's festive to use candy, candied fruits, nuts, cheese balls, and other condiments to decorate the house. They seem to lurk at every corner, and are easy to scoop up as you pass by. Instead, use scented sachets, pine cones, and primitive crafts that are inedible.

"Our family traditionally decorated the tree with candy canes that we eventually ate. Now we string popcorn and cranberry chains."

Ginger, age 51, 30 pounds lost

Gift Giving

A lot of food gifts are passed around this time of year because something homemade is definitely a more meaningful display of affection. But your delicious homemade cookies may not be appreciated by a calorie-conscious recipient. Make an arrangement of dried flowers, a simple pine cone wreath, or framed picture. Not only will it be just as meaningful, but it's a gift that will be a long lasting remembrance.

Portion Control

It's not the food itself that's bad for you, but the excessive portions that are consumed. Having a little of everything is a good way to ensure that nobody's feelings are hurt, and you won't deprive yourself of different tastes.

"Before I head to a holiday party, I have a bowl of high fiber cereal with a large glass of water. It doesn't weigh me down, and yet gives me a sense of control so that I don't eat everything I see."

Mac, age 35, 58 pounds lost

Use Fiber

Bake cookies with added fiber, like oat bran. This will greatly cut the calorie content, and will make the cookie more filling.

Don't Pick

Put your entire meal on one plate so that you know just how much you are eating. Seconds are not an option. Wash it all down with water or a diet beverage. Even better, carry a toothbrush and brush your teeth to indicate to your mind and mouth that you are done.

Buffets

Going to a party that features a buffet can actually be a blessing in disguise. You can survive without the scrutiny that would occur if you were seated. Plus, since you're moving around, the food isn't "in your face" where temptation will be at its full force.

Scan the Table

Look around the buffet table for items that still somewhat resemble the whole foods from which they were derived. Look for dishes based on vegetables, fruits, and grains. Avoid thick sauces and gravy-laden dishes. Fill your plate with fresh vegetables and salads.

Limit Yourself to One Trip

The danger of the buffet is that you may never stop eating. Resolve that you will make one trip, and that you will eat slowly while everyone else is making their third and fourth trip back.

Choose a Small Plate

Take the smallest plate available, and then pile it on. You'll fool yourself into thinking that you're having a big meal. Leave the smallest part of the plate for the food you should have the least of.

Eat Your Favorite Foods First

The food that catches your eye first is the one that

you should eat first. That's the secret of the perpetually thin person.

Go Fish

Shrimp, scallops, crab, and salmon are common buffet fare that are all very low in fat. They'll keep you away from the meatballs and cocktail franks.

Buffet Bites

1. Stick with lean meats or grilled foods.

2. If you love cheese, eat chunks of it and stay away from the spreads.

3. Bean dips contain less calories than sour cream varieties.

4. Salsa is fat-free and a dieter's dream. It usually has only ten calories for two big tablespoons.

5. Choose whole grain crackers over chips.

Pass on the Ordinary

Don't bother to eat what you regularly eat all year. This is the time to enjoy those special foods. Remember this: the first one you eat makes it special. After that, the pleasure is reduced by about 50 percent, and it goes down even further with the third.

Buffet Calorie Count

Buffalo chicken wing = 254 calories
Celery stalk = 6 calories
Cocktail meatball = 20 calories
Whole carrot = 3 calories
Scoop of nuts = 55 calories
Stuffed mushroom = 80 calories
Potato chip with dip = 21 calories
Teaspoon of caviar = 15 calories
One shrimp or scallop = 10 calories
Five Ritz crackers with 1 ounce pate = 200 calories
Three bite-size bacon quiches = 300 calories
Brie in pastry = 230 calories
Eight medium strawberries = 50 calories

Concentrate on People

The fun of a buffet is that it's for mingling, not munching. Move around with a glass of seltzer with lime in your hand and get caught up with the crowd. If you're the hostess, try to have a mingling area that does not involve food. Set up a table with a jigsaw puzzle that all the party goers will attempt to put together.

Low Calorie Party Mix

Oat square cereal
Miniature cinnamon rice cakes
Raisins
Low fat pretzels

Mix together in a festive bowl.

"A great way to prevent a host from bugging me all night to overeat is to take a little bite, and then rave about how delicious the dish is. The reaction is appreciated by the host, and then they move on to somebody else."

Nick, age 67, 38 pounds lost

Alcohol

Those liquid calories can quickly add up. Alcohol is greatly to blame for the extra calories consumed at special events.

Alcohol with Water

Have one glass of water with every glass of alcohol you drink. By alternating between alcohol and water you'll cut your calories in half. Alcohol stimulates appetite, so be aware that as you drink, your willpower will go down.

Watch Those Calories

Research indicates that those alcoholic beverages you're enjoying tonight will turn up as fat tomorrow. These calories are metabolized like fat. There is a way to counteract this effect. By eating magnesium-rich foods like lean cuts of meat, dark green leafy vegetables, and whole-grain products, you will control your body's response to the sugar effect of alcohol. Some people actually take magnesium supplements to normalize their body's response to these sugars when they drink.

Smart Choices

White wine = 80 calories

Light beer = 100 calories

Champagne = 75 calories

Vodka with cranberry juice = 125 calories

Bad Choices

Eggnog = 275 calories

Brandy Alexander = 305 calories

White Russian = 235 calories

Pina colada = 265 calories

Space It Out

If you space out your drinking to one alcoholic

beverage every hour, it greatly cuts down your amount of overindulging not only in alcohol, but it keeps your willpower in check so that you don't overeat.

If You Overdid It

A bartender I know swears this is what you can do that "morning after" you drank too much. Take a shot of vodka, a squirt of lemon, and a drop of Tabasco. Dissolve a beef bouillon in 1/2 cup of warm water. Add it all together, and drink away that hangover.

Valentine's Day

We all know that roses contain a lot less calories than a box of chocolates. But it's okay to indulge from time to time. Here's the calorie count on some of the traditional favorites.

Chocolate candy heart = 69 calories
2 cherry cordials = 180 calories
Candy conversation hearts (1 ounce) = 110 calories

Don't forget the champagne. Two glasses of the sparkly stuff will set you back by only 150 calories. Champagne contains half the calories of sweet wine and one-third the calories of hard liquor. It also aids digestion with its natural carbon gas, magnesium, and potassium.

Easter

Raiding the Easter basket can be dangerous, so dig into those fat-free jelly beans. They are the best sweet in the loot. Each bean contains only about 5 or 6 calories.

Dining Out

Eating in a restaurant can become creative combat

in any diet program. However, with these little steps, it can be a pleasant break from a boring routine without costing a lot of calories.

Don't Arrive Famished

Have a few glasses of water with lemon and a few carrot sticks before heading out.

Save the Alcohol for the Meal

If you enjoy any kind of alcohol when you are dining out, have it during your meal, not before. Alcohol is a high calorie beverage and can stimulate your appetite. It can also impair your judgment about food choices. After all, drinks, especially wines, can enhance the enjoyment of the meal.

Leave Out the Bread Basket

Ask that the breads arrive with the meal, otherwise you'll make a meal out its contents. If you're truly hungry, order an appetizer that takes work to eat. A good choice would be steamed clams or escargot.

Lead the Conversation

Talk a lot during the meal. You can't make polite conversation with your mouth full of food, so let your personality become the table's entertainment.

Diners are most likely to eat foolishly during the first ten minutes of a social gathering.

Cuisine Choices

	Order	Avoid
American	Poultry and seafood	Fatty meats
	Grilled meats	Fried fish
	Vegetables and salads	Dressings
Chinese	Broth-based soups	Fried noodles, egg rolls
	Steamed fish, vegetables	Egg foo yung

189

Chop suey and stir fry	Battered dishes	
White rice	Duck	

French	Steamed mussels	Vichyssoise
	Poached seafood	Quiche
	Seafood/poultry in parchment	Heavy creams (like Remoulade)
	Parfait	Mousse

Greek	Bean and lentil soups	Spanakopita
	Shish kabob	Feta cheese
	Baked fish (Plaki)	Moussaka
	Orzo	Baklava

Italian	Vegetable soup	Antipasto
	Seafood stew (Cioppino)	Fried calamari
	Pasta with vegetables	Pasta with heavy sauce
	Baked or broiled polenta	Marinated vegetables

Mexican	Steamed tortillas	Nachos
	Black and pinto beans	Refried beans
	Salsa	Guacamole
	Gazpacho	Enchilada

Travel

Battling the bulge while traveling is not as difficult as you may believe. It starts when you make your reservations and will make a positive difference in your energy and stress levels. It just takes a little creativity and some advance planning sprinkled in with a little discipline.

Do Some Leg Work

Phone your hotel and ask about gym facilities on site or nearby. Inquire about nearby parks, running tracks, hiking trails, tennis courts, and other exercising options. Ask if there are shuttle services to some of these areas. Even shuttles to shopping areas are good for a spirited mall walk.

Make Reservations

Call your airline and ask about special meals. Every airline will offer an alternative, and your best bet is vegetarian or low fat. Some even offer cold seafood, all fruit, and Hindu (a baked potato and steamed vegetables).

Packing

Tuck a jump rope into your suitcase. You can use it on carpeting or outdoors. Travel with your favorite exercise tape. Hotels that offer convention services will have VCRs that are available for guest use. Pack a pair of walking/running shoes, and fold in an exercise elastic band for resistance work.

At the Airport

Airport delays are frustrating both to the mind and body. Overeating at a food court can result from sheer boredom. Instead, take advantage of the time

Driving

Practice isometrics at traffic lights. Squeeze your buttocks and hold for a count of ten. Raise your lower lip, trying to touch your nose to improve jaw line definition.

191

by walking as fast and as far as you can. If you have lots of "stuff" that would weigh you down, there are convenient lockers located throughout. Some airports have even started installing day gyms.

In the Air

Request an exit row or bulkhead seat. You'll have more comfort and room to move. Take advantage of headphones, and look for the channels with upbeat music. Do some easy leg stretches and move your arms around. Circulation can suffer on long trips.

While in Your Seat

1. Flex your ankles and work your calf muscles.

2. Do seated calf raises with your paperwork (or a child) on your lap.

In the Aisle

1. Grab each ankle and pull your heel up to your buttocks. Hold for a count of ten and alternate.

2. Try to touch your toes while waiting for the lavatory to stretch your hamstrings.

3. Reach up toward the ceiling, alternating hands. Do this ten times.

At Your Hotel

1. Refuse the key to your mini-bar to avoid temptation.

2. Check with your concierge about safe walking or jogging areas.

3. Stage some workouts in the hotel's pool. The natural buoyancy causes the muscles to work harder, and it feels just great.

4. See if your hotel has access to bike rentals.

5. You don't need to pack your weights. Every hotel has books and lamps.

The Mommy Track

It's not necessary to put your diet and fitness routines on hold because there are little ones around. Your kids can help you become more active and fit.

Sports

Find a sport that the whole family can enjoy. Biking (very safe and comfortable models are available) and hiking are sports for kids of every age. Babies love the new running strollers on the market which allow you to power walk/run.

A Natural Weight

Moms get a great upper arm workout by lifting little ones over their shoulders and above their heads.

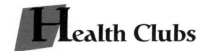

Health Clubs

There's nothing better than an hour reprieve, and you'll be more at ease if you check out gyms and health clubs that offer on site baby sitting services. Separation anxiety? Choose a club where the child center is in your view.

Videos

Check out the video tapes specially created for parent and child bonding.

Chapter Fourteen

Success Stories

Prepare to Get Inspired

Each of the following stories are as different as the people who tell them. Yet there reigns the commonalties of desperation, humiliation, empowerment, and hope.

Out of all the interviews I conducted, I chose only to relate the weight losses with at least a five year longevity. These stories consist of various approaches and rationale. The point of each is that there is a dream that has been fulfilled. I hope that you are inspired, as each of the story tellers inspired me.

Life on the Sidelines

"A tradition at the end of my work day was getting together with my colleagues and chatting about our plans that evening. Although my work as an account manager at an advertising agency was wonderfully fulfilling, and my coworkers were friendly, I couldn't help but feel envious as they would discuss their boyfriends, husbands, and dating plans. All I had to add to the chat was what I was planning for dinner that night and my 'date' with the TV. I was a fat woman, all alone at 33.

Even though they never said anything, I could feel the pity all around me.

"My family moved constantly because of my father's job. At each new school I felt like an outsider, and I comforted myself with food. Of course, that made it harder to make any friends. In high school I would sit on the sidelines while the other girls were asked to dance. So finally, I stopped going anywhere that would add to my humiliation. I stayed home and made friends with my books. By the time I graduated, I was 5´6˝ and 200 pounds.

"In college, I initially lost 30 pounds, probably due to all the excitement and new surroundings. Although I made lots of new friends, the guys on campus looked right through me. At night, while the other girls would go out with their boyfriends, I would stay in my dorm and eat. The weight came right back, along with ten more. I tried a couple

dozen times to diet, but would become discouraged and go off. I can't remember what exactly I ate, mostly fast foods like pizza and subs. I was a secret eater, appearing to eat normally in the cafeteria.

"After college, my twenties became more of the same. Lots of girlfriends (I became a great listener) and no longer concentrating on my books, but on my career. I was promoted to account manager, a prestigious position for someone my age. My extra weight zapped my energy, and at the end of a work day, I would drag home and order out. Usually my choice was Chinese or Italian, or I would pick up something that didn't take a lot of preparation.

"One day at a meeting with some new clients, I saw the most gorgeous man I had ever laid eyes on in my life. He was very nice to me, and I imagined that he was possibly interested. The very thought of seeing him again made me want to do something about my appearance. I wanted to look better just in case there was the possibility that he may have been even slightly attracted to me.

"I started just being aware of everything I ate. For breakfast I would have a small bowl of high fiber cereal with skim milk and fruit, or a bagel and yogurt. At work I'd eat a salad at my desk with a glass of iced tea. Occasionally, I would crave my old favorites like a sub, but now I would eat the filling and not the bread. At night I'd microwave a small box of vegetables and eat the entire thing with lemon and salt and a small portion of fish or chicken.

"First, I noticed that my clothes weren't pulling at me constantly. Then I realized I wasn't always tired. When my coworkers would go out on their dates, rather than feeling sorry for myself I started taking long walks. Because my neighborhood is

not very safe, if it got too dark I would work out to an exercise tape in my apartment.

"After just 5 months, I had lost 45 pounds. By the next client meeting I had dropped my dress size to a 14. I felt good enough about myself to maintain eye contact with this guy. It was fun flirting, and enough to keep me motivated. Three months later I had lost another 25 pounds.

"This time after the meeting he actually asked me to join him for drinks. Although we ended up dating a few times, it didn't work out. But now, I'm dating quite a bit, and when my coworkers get together, I'm right in there, talking about my own dates. I've lost 5 more pounds for a total of 75, and I'm feeling so good about my life that I know I'll never go back."

Marsha, age 33, 75 pounds lost

Food Addict

"As I would reach for the next fattening food, I would ask myself, 'Am I really hungry?' Even if I had eaten an hour earlier, I just couldn't resist. At 5´4˝ I weighed 170 pounds. I wanted every food I saw, and it made me so angry that I had no control. Every day was the dawn of a new diet, and every night I was disgusted with myself for failing.

"Getting an invitation to my tenth high school reunion was the wake up call that gave me the motivation I needed. Even though the event was six months away, I knew that I could not face my classmates 50 pounds heavier than they had remembered me. Two pregnancies and a sedentary lifestyle were no excuse for what my body had become, and I was determined to get back to me.

"I devised a program that I could live with, consuming no more than 1,500 calories a day. I ate five meals a day, consisting of around 300 calories for each meal. The foods that I just couldn't resist, I just didn't bring into the house. I occasionally satisfied my cravings by buying a big cookie or ice cream in the mall. I just didn't bring home a container of it, because I knew that I would end up eating the whole thing.

"I also changed my cooking techniques, broiling meats and chicken, and steaming vegetables and spraying them with cooking spray. If my kids get hungry, I give them fruit and they're just as happy. I know that they'll be healthier by munching on grapes instead of chips, and I won't be guilty of passing along my bad habits.

"Although my husband (also my high school sweetheart) never talked about my weight, I know it bothered him. I lost 40 pounds by my reunion, and I'm trying to lose that final ten. I have more energy, feel younger, and people tell me that I'm nicer to be around."

Pam, age 29, 40 pounds lost

Health Problems

"Being overweight was no laughing matter. The picture of the goodhearted fat guy certainly didn't apply to me. I had constant backaches, shortness of breath, and knee problems that I knew were a direct result of my 100 extra pounds. I had to nap constantly, and my doctor told me that I might need surgery. I knew I couldn't go on feeling so bad.

"Something snapped after seeing an old picture of the 'thin' me. I was at a family gathering, and what I had ignored for so long lay 'staring' at me in the face. I went home and cleaned out my refrigerator. I stopped my love affair with salt and learned to use herbs. I took a 'healthy' cooking course taught by a dietitian and began to exercise. The good news is that my doctor told me that because of the weight loss, I don't need the surgery."

Frank, age 45, 100 pounds lost

Always Big

"I've been bigger than everyone else since I was a child. I never allowed myself to wear 'normal' clothes like jeans and swimsuits. When you're a size 24, you're lucky to find anything, and no way was I going to show my body any more than was absolutely necessary. Doughnuts were my weakness, and I'd go through a box a day. I remember thinking that this is the way God wanted me, and there was nothing I could do.

"Even though I was heavy, I met and married the man of my dreams. He was as nice as I was heavy, and we were very happy. Unfortunately, he was a heavy smoker and became ill with cancer at just 49. When my husband died, I realized that sometimes we can control some of our destiny. Even though I was in deep grief, I didn't want to throw my life away with a food addiction that was equal to my husband's own addiction to cigarettes. Plus, I wanted to enjoy my grandchildren.

"I joined TOPS (Take Off Pounds Sensibly), and at the first meeting I found friends who helped me with both my grief and my weight. Slowly, I lost the weight through learning proper nutrition. It wasn't easy, but rather than turning back to doughnuts when I was hungry or depressed, I would call

a buddy. Now I feel that I'm ready to rejoin life. I have joined a couple of social groups, and although I'm not quite ready to start dating, I know there is something left for me. Plus, my oldest daughter just blessed me with a second grandchild."

Mary, age 54, 135 pounds lost

The Dieting Roller Coaster

"I have had bad eating habits for as long as I can remember. My mother was the neighborhood's favorite baker. Although I was always a little overweight, it never bothered me that much. It wasn't until the summer of my senior year that I decided to make a change. I had been at the beach with some friends when a group of guys stopped by to talk to us. As I walked away, one of them asked my friend if my name was 'Shamu' the whale. I heard the remark, and when I got home, I was shocked to see that I weighed 183 at 5´5˝. I had never been the victim of name calling before, and I was determined never to hear it again.

"Since I was always fairly athletic, I decided to first start walking just 30 minutes a day. The walking slowly turned into running, and somehow I started to lose weight as well as my craving for my mother's baked goodies. I started eating foods that would help my body perform rather than going for the gooey taste.

"By December of my senior year, I had lost over 50 pounds and attended the Christmas Ball wearing a slinky dress in a size seven. The following summer I had lost another 20 pounds, and entered a Miss Hawaiian Tropic contest at a local nightclub and won!"

Tammi, age 20, 70 pounds lost

Stuck in a Chair

"I thought I would die of shame the day I tried to get out a chair and ended up taking the chair with me. I was eating at a restaurant with a bunch of friends. The chair had arms, and since I couldn't fit my 270 pound body into a booth, it was the only seating option. After the meal, I went to get up and found that I was completely stuck. It was absolute humiliation that I will never forget to this day. The entire restaurant filled with stares and snickers.

"After that, just looking at an unhealthy food made me recall that terrible day and how being so overweight differentiated me from everyone else. I can't say I did it overnight, or that I didn't have a few setbacks, but my weight is now 135, just about right for me at 5´7˝. I don't have any particular exercise program except trying to do something to move my body every day. When I go to a restaurant now, I never sit in a chair, because I don't need the memories, and I can very comfortably slide into a booth."

Linda, age 38, 135 pounds lost

New Year's Resolution

"I remember the final new year's resolution that worked. It was the year when I weighed 185 pounds and had one outfit in my closet that fit. I had reached rock bottom. During my teens I played sports, kept active, and my weight was stable at about 130. This kept me in a size 8–10, and seemed right for my height, 5´6˝. But in college, I gained not only the freshman 15, but continued to gain more each year. By the time I graduated, I was almost 190 pounds.

"Somehow I had spaced it all out and still saw myself as that size 10. My denial didn't last, because when I went back home, my niece saw an old picture of me and shouted, 'Boy, you used to be pretty!' My embarrassment and shock at not fitting into any of my old clothing were my keys to sticking to my resolution.

"I lost the weight and have kept it off for six years. In those years I have had two children, a divorce, and experienced the loss of a parent. I don't know why I gained that weight in college. It was probably a combination of loneliness and foods that were different from the type I grew up with. I also believe that the freedom of being able to do and eat anything without thinking about it were factors. I know that going back to the basic food groups along with regaining my active lifestyle were contributors to losing it."

Dee, age 28, 55 pounds lost

Mirrors Don't Lie

"I always thought of myself as a successful business executive who was comfortable with my appearance until one day I caught sight of a sloppy, fat balding man in the mirror of a local department store. When I realized I was looking at myself, it put me into total shock and I couldn't shake the image from my mind. Then one day I interviewed a potential employee who looked like I did when I was younger. Then I found out that he was my age, only 50 pounds lighter. I knew I had finally run out of excuses.

"So what did I do? Like a fool I went home and to eat my last meal. Literally, I ate until I was sick to my stomach. This turned out to be the exorcism that I needed to get started. I ate three meals a day, nothing fancy, but no junk. I lost 7 pounds in the first week, and that pumped me up with confidence to start exercising.

"At first it took me almost an hour to walk two miles. But I kept it up because I finally felt in control. I know this isn't normal, but I lost the 50 pounds in just four months. I feel younger five years later than I have in the last ten years. I can't do anything about the balding, but finally I feel that I've slowed down the aging process, if just a little."

Phil, age 42, 50 pounds lost

Quitting Smoking

"Ten years ago, I decided to quit smoking. My goal was to get healthy, but I was afraid of gaining weight. About a month after stopping the cigarettes and kind of laying low, I started walking and watching what I ate. When I would feel the need to put something in my mouth, I would munch on some baby carrots. I give myself 10 pounds to play with, and the end result is that I'm 38 pounds less than I was when I was a smoker. I've kept the weight off for ten years, except for a 15 pound gain when I broke my leg skiing and I was unable to exercise."

Nick, age 67, 38 pounds lost

"I began smoking when I was in college because all the girls in my sorority smoked. What began as a social habit—smoking when I was drinking to avoid eating—became a pack a day habit. When I met my future husband, he tried to engage me in sports, but I would end up becoming winded. I made the decision to stop smoking, or be left behind.

"Since I was dating a health freak, I changed all of my bad habits. I started drinking water instead of soda, staying away from beer, and eating more fruits and vegetables. Rather than gaining weight from quitting smoking, I was able to run without losing my breath, and the running and better eating habits helped me to go from a size 10 to a 6."

Sara, age 23, 28 pounds lost

Night Eating

"No one ever saw me eating. I ate in secret, when no could judge my food selections or the quantity of my portions. All my life it seemed I never weighed below 160 pounds. People told me I had a pretty face, but it never motivated me to bother to go on a real diet. I would eat for the pure pleasure of it until my stomach hurt.

"I would crawl into bed, just about drunk from the food binge, and then wake up with a major headache. I would look in the mirror, and my face would be so bloated that no matter how much makeup I would apply, I just didn't look or feel pretty. Then I would eat nothing all day while in public and go back to night bingeing.

"When my sister announced that she was getting married, I assumed that I would be the maid of honor, or at least a bridesmaid. When she told me that unless I lost some weight, she wasn't going to include me at all in the bridal party, that became my turning point. I was angry at her, but also at myself. I joined Weight Watchers and lost 7 pounds the first week. Although I really didn't enjoy the meetings, I stayed pretty much on their diet and ended up losing 30 pounds in just six weeks.

"On the day of the bridal party fittings, I was able to fit into a size 10 gown. At 5´5˝, I was still not feeling where I wanted to be, and on the day of the wedding, I had lost another 8 pounds. My gown was really loose, but it only made me proud. Today my weight has evened out at 128."

Mindy, age 30, 32 pounds lost

Never Too Late

"There is not a diet out there that I didn't try. I spent my entire teen years and twenties going up and down the scale by at least 35 pounds. I went to hypnotists, tried diet clubs, and even acupuncture. In my thirties I moved into a neighborhood where everyone socialized at a local fitness club. Since I'd never really exercised to any extent before, I found myself reluctant to join. But being new and alone, I jumped in. It made all the difference in my attitude towards my body.

"Years of dieting had left me flabby, and without a great energy reserve. The sense of belonging and

205

support from my new friends gave me such a 'high' that I began to make exercise a daily routine. We shared friendship, fitness routines, and diet tips. This sharing got me into a sensible routine that has helped me to lose 40 pounds, and become firmer and fitter in my forties than I can honestly say I was in my teens. I have learned that there is no magic pill I can swallow that will substitute for common sense. I admit that it still takes a lot of hard work, but the way I feel now and the body I see in the mirror makes it all worth it.

"I feel good knowing that I can eat foods that will make me look and feel better, and that low fat foods can be made to be as delicious as any of those gooey snacks that I used to crave. I don't like the word 'diet,' because to me, it brings back memories of the torture and deprivation I felt when I went on those crazy gimmicks. I just call it my 'way of living.'"

Margaret, age 47, 40 pounds lost

Starving Myself Fat

"With every diet I went on, I would end up 5 or 10 pounds fatter than when I began. At my lowest point, my highest weight was close to 200 pounds. I tried meal supplements and would feel deprived because I loved to chew. I tried exercise equipment and quickly became bored and out of breath. I had a roomful of stair steppers, thigh machines, and ab rollers.

"A basic couch potato, I suffered from hypertension, and even sex with my husband had become less enjoyable. I knew I had to figure out why I was getting fatter and fatter, so I took myself to a therapist. I found out that I suffered from anxiety and was given medication to cope. But it was the therapy itself that helped me to learn how to handle my anxiety without turning to food to self-medicate. I started a food diary to find out what I was eating and the feelings that led to my food choices.

"I was shocked to learn that I was consuming almost 4,000 calories a day. My goal was to get healthier as well as thinner, and I started planning my meals out. I wrote down what I would eat for the day and stuck with it. Occasionally, I would make substitutions, but tried to keep with the list. Slowly the weight came off. As it did, the anxiety dropped.

"I eventually went off the medication, and ended therapy. I learned that there were other ways to handle stress and anxiety besides quick fixes with comfort foods. I also learned that I had become a caregiver to everyone but myself. My weight loss has given me the confidence to pursue interests I had put on hold because of my weight."

Teresa, age 41, 60 pounds lost

Pregnancy Weight

"I gained a lot of weight with my pregnancies that I never lost. After my third child I decided to get back in shape. I was determined not to be an embarrassment to my children, as my obese mother had been for me. Although I loved my mother dearly, kids would make fun of her, and I was always protective of her. It was a burden no child should have.

"Although I didn't have dreams of looking like a supermodel, I wanted to be able to attend school functions and sporting activities that my kids were in without looking fat and sloppy. I also needed to do it 'my way,' and since money was tight, without a lot of expensive equipment and foods. My program was really very simple. When I was hungry, I made sure that I had something with little or no calories to eat. I had a stockpile of carrots, celery, and rice cakes. If I drank a lot of water, I found that I wasn't as hungry.

"After reading a lot about nutrition, I gave up meat and relied heavily on fish. I made sure all my dairy products were nonfat (I was a 'cream in my coffee' addict), and chose foods, especially cereals, that had a lot of fiber in them. The best part of losing those pregnancy pounds is that my kids are as proud of my weight loss as I am."

Linda, age 42, 38 pounds lost

A Sisterly Bet

"I was raised in a southern town, where we knew one way to cook, and that was deep fat frying. We would even fry our vegetables. Growing up with my twin sister it was never a problem. We were very active, co-captains of our cheerleading squad, and just being active helped us to stay slim.

"After college, we both got married and moved to different parts of the country. I got busy having children, and with my now sedentary lifestyle of changing diapers and washing bottles, the pounds just started to pile on. I avoided mirrors and got into the whole mommy scene without thinking too much about my appearance. I nibbled all day, whenever I was bored or stressed out or watching my favorite program. I couldn't sit down without reaching for something to eat.

"When I cooked, it was the recipes from my hometown: lots of fried chicken, fritters, and even fried eggs. All through my pre-babies years my weight had been around 135. Since I am tall, 5´8˝, this was perfect for me. When I bothered to go near a scale, I saw the pounds slowly creep up to a shocking 190. I was now squeezing into size 16 jeans, and usually didn't bother to try to squeeze since comfort was my main concern.

"My everyday attire became an oversized sweater or tee-shirt, and stretch pants with an elastic band. My day of reckoning came at a special Christmas celebration arranged by my parents. Since money was tight with young children, they decided to spring for airfare for my family and my twin sister's family for some old-fashioned holiday festivities.

"At my parents' home, when my sister and I met eyes, it was like looking into an unflattering mirror. She had gained almost as much weight as I had, which we quickly acknowledged and

bemoaned. We commiserated and waffled between accepting our new lifestyles and wanting to do something about it. Because we had always been somewhat competitive, we decided to make a bet.

"By our next gathering, the one who had lost the most weight would get a day of beauty at a local spa near our home. Even though I had no money to join a gym, I decided that I needed to become more active. I started taking walks after my husband came home each day and could take over with the kids. I joined a play group so that I could have some kind of social life and get away from the boredom grazing I had been doing all day.

"My cooking changed, and I slowly started to cook more simply and without all the fat and oils. When my kids would nap, I would give myself beauty treatments like masks, manicures, and other little treats to make myself feel more feminine. Slowly, the weight started to come off. It took nine months, but I eventually lost 45 pounds. I seemed to level off at that point, and before long it was time for another Christmas celebration.

"This time, because my father's health had been failing, we all paid our own way back home. Although we knew by sight, my sister and I hit the scales to see who had won the bet. My sister had lost 30 pounds, and I had won the bet. Being sisters, we congratulated each other for having both been successful, even though I had lost 15 more pounds. Both of us spent a wonderful day of just being together and getting totally pampered. The competition was good for us, and we have both have kept our weight down for seven years."

Lucy, age 37, 45 pounds lost

Final Motivation

"I developed a herniated disk because I was so overweight. The pain was terrible. The day I was put on a stretcher to the hospital was the day I decided to change my life forever."

Henry, age 66, 135 pounds lost

"I overheard one of my son's kindergarten friends whisper, 'Look how fat Chad's mother is.' I realized my weight didn't just affect me, but could badly affect my child."

Diane, age 36, 70 pounds lost

"One day I got out of the shower, wrapped a towel around me, and was horrified to find that it wouldn't go around my body."

Tina, age 56, 120 pounds lost

"I began wearing only my husband's clothing. They were the only things I could fit into. The look on his face every day made me face my weight problems."

Patricia, age 40, 60 pounds lost

"When I was in college, I took a walking course and couldn't walk up the hill with the rest of the class. I had to stop several times to rest and catch my breath."

Sandy, age 22, 65 pounds lost

"I developed gestational diabetes when I was pregnant, and put my baby at risk because of my weight."

Angie, age 33, 140 pounds lost

"I dated a guy who always made remarks about my weight. My friends confronted me about the verbal abuse I was taking and made me aware of how little I had come to regard myself."

Laurie, age 25, 65 pounds lost

My mailman asked

me when my baby was due, and I wasn't even pregnant. The humiliation of telling him that I wasn't expecting, along with his startled reaction, was the catalyst I needed for finally getting my act together.

Nicole, age 29, 47 pounds lost

211

"I avoided playing sports with my son and preferred being a couch potato. He turned to a friend's dad for interaction which put me to total shame."

Sam, age 39, 80 pounds lost

"I was starting a new job and wanted to make a total change in how I was being perceived as a person. I wanted to be known for my accomplishments, not just my weight."

Paul, age 41, 50 pounds lost

"My husband left me for a thinner woman. She wasn't attractive, younger, or sexier. She even looked like I did when I was thin."

Judy, age 50, 110 pounds lost

"I got stuck in a turnstile in a subway terminal. Three people had to push me through, and the pity and disgust of their looks kept me dieting for an entire year until I lost all the weight."

Frieda, age 43, 160 pounds lost

"I had failed on my fourth weight loss program and it had cost me over $900. I realized that I was the only one could take the weight off my body."

Barbara, age 39, 80 pounds lost

"I saw myself in a three-way mirror at a department store. I didn't realize how fat I had become because I only looked at myself from the waist up."

John, age 32, 30 pounds lost

"Everything I did took too much effort. Even doing my grocery shopping, which was my favorite activity, had left me short of breath."

Linda, age 49, 90 pounds lost

"The doctor told me that I was morbidly obese. Up until then I had always considered myself chubby."

Frank, age 60, 140 pounds lost

Chapter Fifteen

Bargains and Freebies

It's Not Necessary to Spend a Lot to Lose a Lot

As I told you in the first chapter, after conducting hundreds of interviews with successful dieters, there was no correlation between the amount of money spent on dieting and the amount of weight lost. Quite frankly, a large percentage of my interviewees felt that they had wasted the money they had laid out in "promises." Many of them felt betrayed by the hype.

There are wonderful resources available for limited budgets. As you take charge of your weight and your life, consider developing a consumer approach to all the advertising hoopla that preys on our egos. Start by reading labels. If you're looking for supplements, you'll find that the name brands contain the same ingredients as the generic versions. Additional research and effort takes a little extra time, but it will be well worth it. You'll be amazed at the savings.

Vitamin and Diet Supplements

A-1 General Vitamin

P.O. Box 1500
Chapel Hill, NC 27515
1-800-323-8482 (9 a.m. to 5 p.m. ET)

A variety of vitamins, and a flat $2.95 shipping fee.

Discount Natural Foods

2120 Burnet Avenue
Syracuse, NY 13206
1-800-541-1121

Orders are shipped in 24 hours, free of charge. Products include MET-Rx, Creatine, Balance Bars, and Androgen. Specials change every week, and include juicers.

Freeda Vitamins, Inc.

36 East 41st Street
New York, NY 10017
1-800-777-3737

Vitamins, minerals, and nutritional products are offered at savings up to 40 percent. A free catalog is available. It is a lovely, family-owned company, where the founder is a well-known chemist. They'll even provide you with an additional 20 percent courtesy discount just for asking for it.

Vitamin Connection

1-800-760-3020
http://www.vitaminconnection.com

This company has a website for online ordering, or call for a catalog. Supplements sold include St. John's Wort, Creatine, and DHEA.

Vitamin House
1900 Princeton Pike
Lawrenceville, NJ 08648
1-888-882-0708 In NJ: 609-695-5570
http://www.vitaminhouse.com

National top name-brand vitamin and diet supplements like Universal, Ginsana, Kyolic, MET-Rx, Twin Lab, and Weider are sold at savings up to 30 percent.

Vitamin Shoppe
4700 Westside Avenue
North Bergen, NJ 07047
1-800-223-1216

Features 200 brands and 17,000 products. Call for a free copy of their catalog.

Exercise Equipment

Fitness Discount Outlet
1-888-828-FIT-1 (3481)
email: ChampagneFitnessMarketingSales@FIT-1.com

Equipment from Body-Solid Exercise Equipment and Yukon Strength Training Equipment. A large line of fitness and exercise equipment is offered including home gyms, commercial gyms, and free weights. They guarantee they will beat competitors' prices.

Internet Resources

Did you ever dream that you could lose weight by turning on your computer? There is tremendous support waiting for you on the World Wide Web. You can find a dieting buddy, enter a support group relating to your specific problems, and chat with other people just like you. It's anonymous, and you don't even need to leave your home.

"Having someone I can share confessions with has made all the difference in my weight loss. When I'm ready to head for the kitchen because that blueberry pie is calling my name, I turn on the computer. Someone is always there, ready to talk."

Penny, 45, 22 pounds lost

Balance Magazine

http://hyperlink.com/balance
A monthly online magazine on fitness and health.

Calorie Control

http://www.caloriecontrol.org
The official site of the Calorie Control Council. You'll find information on low calorie sweeteners,

fat replacers, trends, and statistics. A lot of invaluable consumer information not available at other sites is here.

Cyber Diet

http://www.cyberdiet.com
Answers your questions about adopting a healthier lifestyle. Information on eating right, exercise, and recipes.

Cyber Kitchen

http://www2.shapeup.org/cyberkitchen
Enter your height, weight, age, and gender, and the amount of exercise you normally do. Then enter your dieting goals, and what you'd like your fat intake to be. You'll receive a daily menu and a plan of action. This website is part of Shape Up America, former Surgeon General C. Everett Koop's campaign for healthy weight and physical

fitness. This site will even provide you with a shopping list for every meal plan.

Diet City

http://www.dietcity.com

This site provides diet tips, book reviews, free diet profiles, BMI measurement tools, and an online weight loss clinic.

Fitness Online

http://fitnessonline.com

Features links to major fitness magazines on the Internet.

Fitness Partner Connection

http://primusweb.com/fitnesspartner

Devoted to providing quality fitness-related information, education, and services. Intent of site is to provide healthy and fit lifestyles.

Good Health Web

http://www.social.com/health

An attempt to bring together valuable information about the field of health.

Healthy Choice Kitchen

http://www.healthychoice.com

A one-stop resource for the calorie conscious. Although it contains some advertising, it gives you lots of great recipes listing calories, fat, sodium, fiber, and vitamin content.

Healthy Ideas

http://www.healthyideas.com

This is the website of *Prevention* magazine, containing personalized meal plans, calculations of calorie intake, as well as easy, low fat recipes. You can actually create your own weight loss program in just minutes with their interactive tools.

Home Arts

http://homearts.com

This is the center for many of the leading magazines. You'll find excerpts from these publications as well as discount coupons and forums where contributors talk about what worked or didn't work in their diet and exercise programs.

Low Fat Lifestyle Forum

http://mardiweb.com/lowfat

This forum is aimed at adopting a low fat lifestyle and diet.

Mayo Clinic

http://www.mayo.ivi.com/mayo/recipe/htm/maintoc.htm

At this site, you'll find more than 200 recipes analyzed and taste-tested by dietitians from the Mayo Clinic. You can also submit a recipe that can be "decalorized" by a registered dietitian.

Men's Fitness Online

http://www.mensfitness.com

The website for the magazine of the same name containing lots of information on fitness, health, sports, sex, etc.

Nutrition Analysis Tool

http://spectre.ag.uiuc.edu/~food-lab/nat

Allows anyone to analyze the foods they eat for various different nutrients.

Shape Magazine

http://www.shapemag.com

The website of the magazine by the same name oriented towards women interested in fitness tips.

Richard Simmons

http://www.richardsimmons.com

This popular diet guru has a delightful site with lots of tips and motivation. If you're one of his many fans, you'll find it absolutely inspirational. Of course there's lots of stuff that he's selling, but Richard's not stingy with his free online goodies

USA Today

http://www.usatoday.com/life/health/lhd1.htm

A chance to catch up on the latest information on diseases and treatments, drugs, and related medical news.

Medical Advice

American Dietetic Association

http://www.eatright.org

The official pages of this important organization where you can email questions to the experts and obtain a researched response. An easily accessible objective source for scientifically-based food and nutrition information.

Carbohydrate Addict's Official Home Page

http://www.carbohydrateaddicts.com

Authors and physicians, as well as successful dieters, the Hellers share information about the correlation between insulin imbalance and obesity.

Heart Information Network

http://www.heartinfo.org

An independent, educational website that provides a wide range of information and services to heart patients and others interested in learning about lowering risk factors for heart disease.

Intelihealth

http://www.intelihealth.com/ih/ihthome

A collection of consumer health information and answers to personal medical questions by experts. Also contains information about common health issues in conjunction with Johns Hopkins University.

The Science of Obesity and Weight Control

http://www.loop.com/~bkrentzman

An award winning website containing the best links to scientific obesity information on the web.

Weekly Internet Support Groups

There are live chat groups on the Internet that meet weekly. The support these live forums project is palatable. It's real people talking about their lives and dieting dilemmas without fear of judgment. This is just a sampling. Check out the chat areas of your Internet provider to find even more. The following chats take place at http://www.thriveonline.com, or AOL Keyword "thrive".

Monday 8 p.m. ET
Battling the Bulge

Tuesday 8 p.m. ET
Battling the Bulge

Wednesday 8 p.m. ET
Battling the Bulge

Thursday 8 p.m. ET
Battling the Bulge

Friday 8 p.m. ET
Battling the Bulge

Saturday 8 p.m. ET
Collegiate Battle of the Bulge

Sunday 10 p.m. ET
Weight Loss Buddies

Health and Fitness Newsgroups

The Internet has newsgroups, similar to bulletin boards, linking you to people with common dieting and fitness interests. Just post your question or dilemma, and keep checking back for replies. Your ability to access these groups depends on your Internet access provider. Here are some popular newsgroup addresses to check out:

Fitness and Health

alt.meditation
alt.sport.weightlifting
alt.yoga
misc.fitness.aerobic

misc.fitness.misc
misc.fitness.walking
misc.health.alternative
misc.kids.health

Food and Nutrition

alt.food.fat-free
alt.food.low-fat
sci.med.nutrition

Sports

alt.mountainbike
alt.rec.camping
rec.running
rec.sport.tennis
rec.sport.swimming
rec.sportunicycling

These are just a few of the news groups available. You can use your browser to find several that relate to your specific interests. If your server doesn't provide a newsgroup browser, use a web search engine like Yahoo (http://www.yahoo.com) or Deja News (http://www.dejanews.com).

Cooking on a Budget

Do you think you can't lose weight because you can't afford the expensive, healthier food choices? If you're on a fixed income and can't afford to purchase fresh produce and prepackaged diet foods, there are lots of healthier, cheaper alternatives.

Pasta

Stock up on different varieties. Don't bother with expensive, fattening prepared sauces. Combine pasta with a simple can of tomatoes, or a little olive oil and cheese. Pasta is as unlimited as your imagination. Experiment with various tastes.

1. Top pasta with leftover vegetables and meats.

2. Use soup broths to flavor up plain pasta.

3. Add reduced-fat mayonnaise and vinegar to pasta salad.

4. A small amount of herbs can replace sauce in many pasta varieties.

5. Use leftover chicken and chicken bouillon cubes to moisten and reflavor.

Beans

Use beans to stretch out a meal. Not only will you save money, but beans contain vitamins that make your eating more healthy. Add beans to extend hamburger.

Oatmeal

It's cheap, it's high fiber, and it's a great extender! Oatmeal is an inexpensive "comfort" food. Add a cup of oatmeal to many of your favorite recipes. It will make any cookie recipe more healthy for you and your family. Trust me, they won't notice the difference. It's also one of the best extenders around for meat loaf.

Meats

Check out some of the cheaper cuts of meat at your supermarket. They contain less fat, and if cooked with a little bit of creativity, are much tastier. When cooking with poultry, purchasing the thighs is a much cheaper choice than breast meat. It takes just a few extra minutes to debone the meats yourself. Purchasing anything that is boneless is a luxury that is just not worth the price if you're on a budget.

Exercise on a Budget

Maybe you can't afford to join an expensive gym or class, or buy overpriced home equipment. People have been exercising long before the

Soups

It doesn't take a gourmet chef to make soup from scratch. Just heat up some puréed vegetables and use broth and apple juice to thin it to the consistency you want. Season it with cinnamon and nutmeg. It's a great way to sneak veggies into your diet.

advent of any these mechanical means, maybe even doing better without them.

Videos

1. Tape your favorite exercise program from the many on TV today. Use it repeatedly.

2. Use your library and rent tapes. You'll never be bored. There are over 300 fitness videos on the market today, so your local library should have a good selection.

Walking/Running

It's free, and it's one of the best overall workouts. Choose and vary scenic routes to prevent boredom.

Housework and Gardening

You'll save money on landscapers and house-keepers when you do it yourself. Plus dieters report that there's an enormous sense of self-gratification. Some would-be exercisers don't join gyms and clubs because they feel that it's a waste of time and money. Become your own personal trainer by putting a little more steam into regular daily activities.

1. While vacuuming, do some lunges.

2. When pulling on those pesky weeds, bring your arms back to get rid of that "jiggle" and tone the underarm area.

3. Tone arms and whittle that waist by pressing down and twisting your body while mopping and sweeping.

4. Rather than bending at the waist to pick up around the house, do squats.

5. Do stretches when reaching into the kitchen cabinet.

6. Shoveling snow is a great workout.

7. Use two rags when doing hands and knees cleaning and use vigorous circling motions.

8. Use a rotary lawnmower to cut your grass.

9. When unloading and loading the dishwasher, do deep squats.

10. Use broad strokes when raking the yard.

Renting Exercise Equipment

Since studies indicate that over 50 percent of exercise equipment purchases lay unused, it makes good sense to rent. Before making that major investment, try out that stair stepper, treadmill, etc., for a month to see if you really like it and will stick with it. If you decide to keep the equipment, your rental fee is usually applicable to your purchase. Check the Yellow Pages under "Exercise Equipment" or "Rentals." Monthly fees are typically in the $35 to $50 range.

Organizations

Believe it or not, there are diet clubs out there that really exist only to help you lose weight without taking your money. If you can't find one in your area, consider getting a few friends together and starting your own group. If you can't recruit any one you know, put up a notice on your grocery store's community board.

The Net Loss Club

http://www2.itw.com/~thinker/home.html
Founded by Kathy Kramer of Pennsylvania in 1995, this organization sprouted from Kathy's search to find an email diet buddy to share her struggle losing weight. Uses email to offer support and inspiration to over 300 members worldwide.

Overeaters Anonymous

This is a completely nonprofit organization started

in 1960 by three women in Los Angeles to help each other to overcome their eating problems. The program is patterned after Alcoholics Anonymous. There are no dues or fees, but many of the chapters "pass the hat" at meetings in order to cover expenses. There are no "weigh-ins" and no scales to intimidate. Check the white pages of your telephone directory for a location near you.

TOPS

"Take Off Pounds Sensibly" (TOPS) is a nonprofit national group founded in 1948 by Esther Manz, an overweight housewife, in the kitchen of her Milwaukee, Wisconsin home. TOPS helps the overweight attain their weight goals through group support. They usually require a physical examination (with proof). Membership fees are $16 annually for the first two years ($20 in Canada), and $14 annually after that ($18 in Canada). There are also local dues, which are set by each chapter. Normally, they're less than $5 a month. To find out if there's a location near you call TOPS at 1-800-932-8677.

Chapter Sixteen

Other Weight Loss Options

Beyond Dieting

There are options in losing weight that go beyond cutting down on calories. Sometimes dieting and exercise alone cannot engender total satisfaction in one's body. There are techniques that are considered short cuts and final solutions. Some are controversial, while others are risky.

Liposuction

The number one requested cosmetic surgery procedure today is liposuction, the suctioning of excess fat from certain areas of the body. Certain body types carry pockets of fat that just can't be exercised off. It is a procedure that has only been around since the early eighties. When it was originally introduced, the fluid that was extracted was about half fat and half blood. Now, there are new, safer methods that remove almost 100 percent fat alone. Still, it is the informed patients who report the best results. Cosmetic surgery is still major surgery.

Risks

There are very rare reports of complications that can come from any surgery. They include infection, blood clots (sometimes fatal), reactions to anesthesia, or perforation to the skin or organs caused by improper probing or excess force. This is the result of excessive instrument force by inexperienced surgeons.

Candidates
An ethical surgeon will not perform liposuction as a weight loss alternative. The ideal candidate for liposuction should be near a healthy weight for their body type and age.

Who Performs Liposuction?
Liposuction techniques are now being performed by dermatologic surgeons, cosmetic surgeons, and plastic surgeons. Both dermatologic surgeons and plastic surgeons are currently being taught liposuction during their residency training programs.

Body Areas
The most frequently treated areas are the waistline, abdomen, inner and outer thighs (saddlebags), buttocks, knees, ankles, and neck area. Men are now getting liposuction in the breast area.

Ultrasonic Liposuction
This technique uses sound waves to liquefy the fat. The procedure is less invasive than traditional liposuction, making recovery time a lot quicker. Many surgeons are even performing this procedure in their offices or in an ambulatory surgery center. With this procedure, blood loss is greatly reduced.

Gastric Surgery
Surgery to treat chronic or severe obesity grew out of the results of operations for cancer and severe ulcers. It removes large portions of the stomach or small intestine. The result was that these

procedures resulted in large weight losses following the surgery. Surgeons, recognizing the results, began using it to treat patients with a lot of weight to lose as long as 40 years ago. Patients are not considered for this operation unless they are at least 100 pounds overweight or have a body mass index (BMI) of 40 or above. A weight problem must be severe, or even life-threatening, to be considered.

How It Works

The surgery limits how much the stomach can hold. The patient is able to make better food choices and experience satiety that may not have been able to be assuaged previously. Food intake is restricted because for most people the ability to eat a large amount of food is gone. Usually, only one-half to a whole cup of food can be eaten at one time without severe discomfort.

Risks

A small percentage of patients required follow-up surgery to correct complications. Abdominal hernias were the most common complication, but also included were breakdown of the staple line and stretched stomach outlets. Some patients had problems with gallstones. This was the result of losing weight rapidly, which can occur with any quick weight loss.

Other problems included nutritional deficiencies such as anemia, osteoporosis, and metabolic bone disease. These problems are preventable if vitamin and mineral supplements are taken after surgery. A small percentage of the patients had a problem with vomiting. This was caused by overstretching of the stomach by food particles that had not been chewed thoroughly. Less than 1 percent of complications resulted in death.

Success Rate

Research reports that about 30 percent of patients are able to get to a normal weight after this surgery. About 80 percent of patients achieved some degree of weight loss. The problem with this surgery is that some patients are unable to adjust their eating habits. Some surgeons require behavior modification follow-up on their patients. The real success reported by this type of operation was a commitment to a lifelong change in eating and long-term medical monitoring. This is a complicated procedure, only to be used as a profound last measure, and should be carefully researched.

Body Lifts

These are "face lifts" for the thighs, buttocks, hips, and stomach. The procedure smoothes and tightens sagging skin that has lost its elasticity, many times due to excess weight loss.

How It Works

A section of the skin is removed (sometimes after liposuction), and a section of the fibers and muscles beneath it are tightened. The remaining skin is pulled taut and stitched together. Sometimes it is the only way to get rid of cellulite for good.

Cons

Extensive scars are the biggest disadvantage to this type of operation. It's also very expensive, and about five times more costly than liposuction. Since it's major surgery, the risks involving anesthesia, etc., also exist. In some cases, a blood transfusion may be necessary. Recovery time is also somewhat lengthy.

Other Weight-Related Surgeries

Tummy Tuck

This surgery removes excess fat or skin that may have been stretched by pregnancy or obesity. It is performed under general anesthesia and involves several days of hospitalization. There is also an extensive recovery period of several weeks. After a lot of weight is lost, successful dieters may be thrilled with their new bodies, but not their sagging tummy area. My interview subjects reported wanting this procedure first and foremost after their weight loss.

Breast Implants

Due to weight loss, aging, and breast feeding, breast augmentation is being done with saline and

Breast Reduction

Women who are at a normal weight sometimes still felt fat with large breasts. Although losing the weight was a liberating experience, they still reported physical limitations and discomfort caused by oversized breasts. This surgery held the highest satisfaction rate of any of the procedures.

231

occasionally soy bean implants. Silicone breast implants are now illegal in the United States.

Breast Lift

Another surgery that many times follows weight loss. A breast lift raises and shapes droopy breasts. There is some visible scarring from this surgery.

Male Breast Reduction

This is a little talked about operation. Many times excessive breast tissue in men can be reduced with liposuction. Sometimes, although the breasts in men are not bigger, it can appear that way as a result of a large weight loss. In this case, the surgeon will remove the excess skin.

Cellulite Treatments

I have been witness to the thinnest person dieting away in an attempt to get rid of cellulite. Cellulite is hereditary, and it is not necessarily the result of heavy legs and thighs. I've seen 90 pound anorexic models with cellulite. There are many treatments available today, most of them can be used at home.

Acids

There are a myriad of acid-based creams on the market today. The acids speed up natural exfoliation, making dimply skin look smoother. Look for percentages in the 12 to 15 percent range. Or to get a natural acid without the chemicals, use milk. Powdered milk is lactic acid. Make a thick paste by adding a little water to the powder and massage it into the affected area. Use a rough washcloth or a loofah, as it's half the art of the massage that works on cellulite.

Caffeine

The way caffeine gets us up and going in the morning is the same way it gets those pesky fat cells going. It's the number one ingredient in some of the priciest cellulite creams available today. Save lots of money by doing this spa treatment yourself. Take your warm, used coffee grounds out of your coffee maker. Sitting on the edge of your bathtub with some newspaper underneath to prevent a mess, rub the grounds into your cellulite. Massage it in thoroughly for at least 5 minutes. Wrap your thighs and the coffee residue with plastic wrap. Let it sit and detoxify the skin for at least 10 minutes. Then just rinse it off. You can also use seaweed (found dried in health food stores) and wet it down as an effective wrap. The seaweed will detoxify the skin and draw out any impurities.

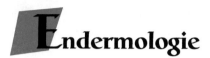

A mechanical massager, available only at endermologie centers, is being used to smooth out skin. The concept is that this machine will draw out the cellulite, knead it, and break up the connective fibers. This procedure is costly, and has to be kept up. Usually it's necessary to have this treatment performed on a weekly basis.

233

Chapter Seventeen

Shortcuts

Fit and Fabulous, Fast!

There are the tricks of the trade used by the best bodies around that work quickly and effectively. They are the techniques that come out when time is of the essence. These are the secrets whispered by trainers, agents, and the stars themselves that are the very cutting edge of the industry. By using these little secrets, you'll be amazed at the results.

The Ultimate Jump Start Diet

The Garlic and Papaya Diet

This is a totally natural diuretic when you need to get into an outfit quickly and safely. Many models use it to prepare for a photo shoot This is the "secret" formula behind very expensive capsules being sold in Hollywood.

Take two garlic tablets and two papaya tablets before breakfast, lunch, and dinner. These tablets are available in your local drugstore or health food store. Ask your pharmacist for the strongest strength available over-the-counter. Eat lightly for two days, staying away from salt, bread, and carbonated beverages. Stay near a bathroom because this will draw fluids (safely) from your body.

Ice Water

Ask anybody with a body "to die for," and most likely they will tell you that they drink lots of water. The water is true, but it's only half the story. It's the ice that you add to your water that really makes the difference. Drinking ice water forces your system to rev up your metabolism, keeping the body's temperature from dropping. For example, if you drink eight 12-ounce glasses of ice water a day, your body will burn an additional 200 calories.

Drink water consistently throughout the day. By the time you are really feeling thirsty, you are on your way to becoming dehydrated.

Often what we think of as hunger is thirst. If you find it difficult to down water in large quantities, flavor it up with a bit of lemon or lime. Water can provide a feeling of fullness, and it helps the kidneys and liver do their job.

Don't be fooled into thinking that drinking lots of water will bloat you. Water retention is more likely to be caused by not drinking enough.

Spicy Foods

Scientists have discovered that chili, peppers, salsa, mustard, and ginger can actually raise your metabolic rate. The result is you can burn calories much faster, up to 45 percent faster than that of a bland diet. How? These foods create a thermogenic burn, meaning it helps the body to produce "heat," thus burning off calories. Forget all those "thermogenesis" products out there. Just start adding some "spice" into your diet.

Say It with Soy

Adding soy to your diet will add more than just a fabulous figure. Soy is packed with powerful antioxidants which interfere with free radical damage. This is the basis for how fast we age. Soy is another reason to turn to a more vegetarian-based diet. Unlike animal proteins, soybeans don't spew scads of damaging free radicals through your body to age your cells. Soy also prevents heart disease and diabetes. Japanese, who eat the most soybean in the world (thirty times more than Americans), live longer than anyone. Soy is also reported to cut breast cancer rates and lower blood cholesterol.

Seeds

To maximize your intake of nutrients, add a lot of seed-containing fruits and vegetables such as apples, pears, and bananas, as well as the seeds themselves (like sesame or sunflower seeds). Seeds are a great source of fiber, allowing foods to go through your body quickly.

237

Look Buff!

Before you shower or bathe, dry brush your body with a coarse loofah. It will slough off dead cells, stimulate circulation, and aid lymphatic drainage. It will unbloat your body!

Tack a Mirror on It

You can purchase a mirror that attaches to the front of the refrigerator. You'll find that if you have to face yourself each time you peek in, it just may wake you up to reality.

Tape up an Inspirational Note

Make that note a trigger for your success. Try something like, "I can do it." or "Just a month until swimsuit season."

Keep the Fat in the Frig

Take one pound of butter or shortening and keep it in a plastic bag. Make it the first thing you see when you open that refrigerator.

Portion All Your Foods

Pack all your food in bags. You'll see your daily allotment at a glance. Knowing that you're limited to those bags provides a focus.

Good Foods for Great Looks!

Blueberries

Promote healthy collagen for fewer wrinkles and help create less constriction of veins and faster healing.

Carrots

Contain high levels of beta carotene for protection against sun damage.

Salmon
Rich in essential fatty acids to keep skin moisturized.

Eggs
High in the amino acid "cystein," necessary for the growth and maintenance of the body's tissues.

Yams
Rich in vitamin A to protect the skin from environmental damage.

Mushrooms
Rich in selenium, an antioxidant that may help lower skin cancer risks.

Yogurt
Contains vitamin B complex, which is essential for smooth, blemish-free skin.

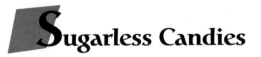

Sugarless Candies

Candies and gums sweetened with

artificial sweeteners can't be broken

down the body efficiently and can

cause severe bloating.

Consider This!

Red Wine
Drinking a glass of red wine can speed up metabolism rates.

Lollipops
Sucking on a lollipop can calm nerves and stop sugar cravings.

Stomachs Can Shrink
After a period of restricting calories, the stomach's capacity will actually decrease.

Tensing
No need to stay at home with an expensive ab machine when you can tense your stomach muscles in and out wherever you are!

The Fat Test
If you want to know if a food is high in fat, but the box isn't around so you can read the labeling, rub the food with a paper napkin. If it leaves a grease mark, it's probably got more fat than you want.

Grow Up!
Start experimenting with exotic foods which are low in calories. For instance, portabello mushrooms are exotic and look like a large steak. Leave those big fat-filled cheeseburgers to the little kids.

Cut Back on Calories without Counting

Eat Your Treats
If you don't treat yourself now and then, you'll just crave it more. It will lead to an unfortunate binge.

Leave Out the Fat

Chances are many of your favorite foods can remain in your diet if you cut back on cheese, butter, cream, etc.

Spread It

Salad dressings, spreads, etc., can be thinned out with vinegars, yogurt, and other low fat extenders.

Check Portions

Weigh and measure your foods when it's convenient.

Stop Late Night Eating

Your body can't digest those late night snacks when it's at rest.

Don't Drink Calories

Learn to like low calorie drinks for painless calorie cutting.

What's in Your Coffee?

Since there are so many specialty coffees around, be certain that you're really ordering a potentially delicious, refreshing low calorie drink.

American drip	4 calories
American decaf	4 calories
Espresso	5 calories
Latte	60 calories
Cappuccino	40 calories
Cafe mocha	150 calories

Don't Skip Meals

You'll end up eating twice as much and your metabolism will be messed up with low blood sugar levels.

Shop with the Right Attitude

Never go shopping for food when you're ravenous! You'll end up with all the wrong stuff in your cart.

Proteins for Weight Loss

All proteins are not the same. To lose weight more quickly, eat egg whites, steamed or grilled fish, chicken, and turkey.

Eating as Meditation

Increase your satisfaction by slowing down and stepping inside of yourself. Remove any distractions, focus on your food, and take only what you need. Chew with deep awareness, noting how you feel when you have finished.

Chew Hard

Any fruit or vegetable that is hard to chew delivers better fiber and prevents blood sugar dips.

Trick Your Body

We all want to sin a little, so stay away from the "all or nothing" syndrome. Replace sugary or fatty snacks with complex carbohydrates and low percentages of fat. No fat foods adds up to no satisfaction.

Sleep More

Studies show that when people don't get enough sleep, they eat more food, and they eat it more often.

Eat It Cold

Foods that are cooled down lose some of their calories and are harder to digest.

Stay Away from Alligators

If a fruit or vegetable has hard skin, it's likely to be higher in calories and fat than smooth skinned varieties. The reason is its water content. That's why a tomato has a lot less calories than an avocado.

Grate Your Food

Use a grater, and watch your food grow. Carrots, apples, and cabbage will really expand when you put them into a food processor.

Refrigerate Cans

By putting your canned meats, soups, gravies, and other canned foods containing fat in the refrigerator, you'll save calories. The fat will collect and rise to the top so you can scrape it off.

Chapter Eighteen

Questions

Most Frequently Asked Questions

Wherever I go, there seems to be a consistency to the questions that I am asked. The following is a compilation of your dieting and exercise questions, and the answers I have researched to the best of my ability.

What is lower in fat, margarine or butter?

Both margarine and butter contain 11 grams of fat per tablespoon. The difference is that the fat in margarine is mostly polyunsaturated, while the fat in butter is saturated. Eating a diet high in saturated fat increases the risk of heart disease and high blood pressure.

How can I prevent my child from developing an eating disorder?

If your child is a picky eater, lay off, and let her pick. Teach your child that people come in all shapes and sizes, and that remarks about weight are unacceptable. Make sure that you set a good example with your own eating habits.

How can I talk to my wife about her weight?

You don't need to talk to your wife about her problem. She already knows she's overweight. You need to get her moving without being obvious. Ask her to take a walk, or offer to cook a meal and make it low fat. Show her a lot of affection and support, and more than likely she will bring up the subject herself.

Is it true that lipstick contains calories?

Get ready to be shocked. The average woman consumes up to nine pounds of lipstick over the course of a lifetime.

How do I know if I need calcium supplements?

If you aren't getting enough calcium from foods, are a smoker, or are on the Pill, chances are that you do need a calcium supplement. It is best absorbed if taken in doses of 500 milligrams or less.

How do I stop my constant eating?

Chances are you're eating out of boredom rather than hunger. You need to find alternatives to eating, like a sport or a hobby. You might need to make some new friends to keep you busy. Eat often to keep your energy up, but not more than six times a day.

Is it better to eat before or after I exercise? I've heard that it is better eat before so that you can work off the calories.

All experts agree that a calorie is a calorie no matter when you use it. They also concur that it's most important to eat when you're less likely to overeat. Also, some people feel shaky when they work out on an empty stomach, while others feel sluggish working out on a full one. A pre-workout snack might be the best bet.

I enjoy appetizers, but most are so fattening. Are there any low calorie choices on the menu?

Stay away from nachos, mozzarella cheese, and those blooming onions. Order a vegetable platter, shrimp cocktail, or best of all, portabello mushrooms.

Is it true that celery actually contains negative calories?

The truth is there's no such thing as negative calories, but celery is one of the lowest calorie foods you can eat, at only six calories a stalk.

Will eating meat prevent me from losing weight?

Meat has great nourishment value, but you need to limit your portions. Even the leanest cuts of meat still contain some fat.

Am I losing nutrients if I switch to skim milk?

Actually, quite the opposite. Skim milk is higher in calcium and protein than whole milk. The only downside is getting used to the flavor. Gradually adding it to your diet will help make it taste less "watery."

How can I tell if a food is fattening if there's no labeling?

You can tell by taking just a bite. If it coats your tongue, your teeth, the back of your mouth, or makes your lips feel slippery, it's probably high in fat.

How can I keep from feeling so deprived when I exercise?

You need to think of exercise as adding to whatever you like to do, rather than subtracting. For instance, if you like TV, buy a treadmill and watch it while you exercise.

Besides coffee, is there anything that I can do at work to get rid of that mid-afternoon slump?

Revive tired muscles and stimulate blood flow by placing a plastic water bottle on the floor. Take off your shoe and gently roll your foot over it from your heels to your toes. Repeat with the other foot. This reflexology technique will pep you right up!

Are there any foods that can give me more stamina?

Choose proteins for more long-term energy. Meats and low dairy products will take longer to digest.

Does salt really cause water retention?

Too much salt in the diet not only causes puffiness in the face and body, but it can lead to health troubles in later years.

Isn't a craving just telling me what my body needs?

If that was so, you'd be craving a lot more spinach and whole grains. Most of the time, a craving is just wishful thinking or a need for something comforting (comfort foods).

Are the "natural" diet pills sold in health food stores really safe?

Not if they contain ephedrine (ma-huang). Overdoses of this herb have been reported to cause rare cases of stroke, seizure, heart attack, and even death.

Is it true that toast has fewer calories than bread?

No, toasting bread, bagels, or other breads does nothing to alter its chemistry. The calorie content remains the same.

Why do plateaus occur in dieting?

Plateaus usually happen after a dieter has been dieting for some time. The real reason is that after some weight is lost, dieters need to drop their calorie allowance or increase their exercise even further to allow for further weight loss. Making this adjustment seems to get the weight moving again.

Is it possible to speed up metabolism?

The best way to increase metabolism is to increase muscle mass. Muscle requires more energy to maintain than fat. The more body fat, the harder it is to lose weight.

Is there any way to lose weight in a certain area of the body?

Unfortunately, there's no way to predict where weight will be lost. Spot reducing is a myth, and it's not even possible to spot reduce by exercising. There are certain body types that are earmarked by genetics.

How can I stay motivated throughout my diet?

Motivation seems to suffer when dieters make unrealistic goals and demands on their bodies. This results in discouragement and backsliding. Keep goals realistic, and allow for a few minor setbacks.

Should I stop working out if I'm sore?

Some soreness is natural when exercising. Usually getting moving again will make it feel better. If it doesn't stop in a day or two, cut back a little bit. However, if it's actually pain that you're experiencing, stop exercising. Ice the joint, and if it doesn't heal in a few days, see a doctor.

How do I get enough calcium in my diet if I don't eat dairy products?

There is calcium in dark green leafy vegetables. Unless you're eating five servings of these a day, you should take a calcium supplement.

Is sugar really bad for you?

Too much sugar in a diet is not conducive to weight loss because it's immediately turned into reserve fat. It's also a factor in diabetes and hardening of the arteries, often found in the obese.

Is there any difference in olive oil, peanut oil, sunflower oil, and safflower oil?

No, they all contain the same calories, about 120 per tablespoon.

I know it's important to dring eight to ten glasses of water a day. Does diet soda count?

Yes, as long as the soda is decaffeinated. Caffeine is a diuretic and can cause dehydration. The purpose of drinking fluids is to hydrate the body. However, diet soda can cause bloating, so water is still your best bet.

251

Is it nutritionally sound to occasionally substitute cereal for a meal?

Whole grain, vitamin-fortified cereals with fruit are a great quick meal that can be substituted for lunch or dinner if the rest of the day's menu is balanced.

Does muscle really weigh more than fat?

Absolutely! A one pound slab of fat weighs just one pound, obviously. However, that same amount of fat would weigh 22 percent more as muscle, because muscle is more dense.

Is it true that you can eat certain foods in combination with other foods to burn calories more efficiently?

Every scientist and expert I questioned on this came up with same answer, NO! They tell me it makes absolutely no biological sense. Furthermore, it goes against all scientific knowledge of body chemistry and digestion.

Is it true that I increase my risk of diabetes if I'm overweight?

At least 80 percent of people with diabetes were overweight at diagnosis. So it is true that maintaining a healthy weight will reduce the risk of developing diabetes. If you have diabetes, losing weight can help bring blood sugar levels to more normal levels and reduce risk of diabetic complications.

What is the normal amount of weight gained just before menstruation?

According to most gynecologists, the range of normal weight gain is from 1 to 4 pounds. Any more weight gained is due to dietary changes (PMS cravings).

How do I figure out how many calories a day to eat in order to lose weight?

You need to consume 15 calories per pound of body weight. No more than 30 percent of those calories should come from fat. Realistically a good target calorie count is around 1200 calories on average. Any less is too difficult to maintain for a long period.

Can I still eat cheese and lose weight? I've heard that it's one of the worst foods for losing weight.

If you love cheese, and can't live without it, choose varieties that are softer in texture. Eating bread or fruit with the cheese will fill you up more quickly.

What are good protein sources if I've decided to give up all meats including chicken and fish?

Low fat dairy products, beans, rice, peanut butter, and tofu are all excellent replacements if you've decided to alter your diet in this manner.

Do fruit juices contain any fiber?

They contain no fiber at all. Eat the fruit itself if you're looking for a good fiber source.

Is it all right to still include wine with my meals if I'm trying to drop a few pounds?

Yes, you can still have wine if you remember to count it as part of your meal. A good way to do this is to substitute a slice of bread, or take about 70 calories away from your meal.

What is a good low fat treat to have after dinner?

Try a little diet Jell-O with a dollop of whipped cream on top, or eat a couple of marshmallows. Both these choices will set you back a mere 10 to 20 calories.

I can't watch a movie without munching on something. Any ideas?

A lot of dieters reported that instead of high fat concession stand popcorn, they brought in a bag of cereal, like Kellogg's Corn Pops. These cereals provide that crunchy, sweet satisfaction without the fat.

What has more health advantages, stationary cycling or regular bicycling?

They provide equal health benefits, but the former can be truly boring unless you can read or watch a program to make up for the loss of scenery.

How many different foods should I eat at a meal?

Dieters found that if they had too many choices at a

meal, they were more likely to overeat. Giving yourself no more than three items at a time provided the right variety and nutrition.

Is there any way to trim down my favorite food, pizza?

If you order your pizza with a thin crust, and with little or no cheese, you can make a nutritious meal. Ask for extra vegetables like mushrooms and onions, and leave off the pepperoni. It contains too many calories.

What are the biggest dieting gimmicks around today?

Oh gee, where do I start? There's those patches that you apply to your skin that promise to melt fat while you sleep. Oh yes, and don't let me forget those creams and lotions that promise to reduce

Is it true that light mayonnaise is still high in fat?

Even light mayonnaise gets 75 percent of its calories from fat. If it's mayo's slightly sour flavor you love, mix one cup of plain nonfat yogurt with one tablespoon of mustard.

255

inches. There seems to be something new popping up every day. If it advertises "working overnight" or "melt fat in minutes" stay away. Hey, did you hear the one about the breath spray that curbs all your food cravings?

If I eat a cereal with raisins, how much do I need to equal a serving of fruit?

A normal one ounce serving of cereal with raisins contains less than 1/4 cup. It would take about three servings of cereal to get a full serving of fruit, so you'll need to add more raisins, or for a lower calorie count, blueberries.

I understand that potatoes are a good diet choice, but what size is a serving?

A small potato, about the size of your fist, or four inches long is about a serving.

Chapter Nineteen

Recipes under 200 Calories

Enjoy Your Favorite Foods!

The recipes in this chapter are real food! These are recipes that you would be absolutely proud to serve your family and friends. I have also intentionally chosen recipes that are easy to make, with products that are readily available.

I encountered lots of difficulty while researching recipes for this chapter. Many recipes that were allegedly "slimming" were anywhere from 500 to 600 calories. That's not a diet recipe to me. Other recipes had as many as 20 to 25 ingredients. If you're like me, you would not attempt to cook with that many steps. Our lives are just too busy, and we're too hungry to wait! After the fifth ingredient, I'm out the door to the nearest fast food outlet. What you'll love about this chapter is that each of the recipes are a cinch to make, and absolutely delicious! Plus, you can mix and match until you get the number of calories you'd like to consume for any particular day.

I've tried to include something for everyone's taste. The last thing I would do is tell you to eat cauliflower if you hate it. There are also some low fat desserts for those of us who just can't end a meal without a "little something" sweet. Trust me, your family will not know the desserts are low fat, and neither will your taste buds.

Enjoy!

Appetizers and Dips under 200 Calories

Hot Spinach Artichoke Dip

95 calories per serving
Makes 24 servings

1 cup grated Parmesan cheese
1 cup low fat mayonnaise
1 can (14 ounces) artichoke hearts, drained and chopped
1 package chopped spinach, thawed and drained
2 tablespoons tomato
Garlic, salt, and pepper to taste

Heat oven to 350 degrees. Mix all ingredients, except tomato. Spoon into 9-inch plate or quiche dish. Bake 30 to 35 minutes or until lightly browned. Serve topped with chopped tomato.

Stuffed Mushrooms

41 calories per serving

Makes 4 servings

12 large mushrooms

2 tablespoons lemon juice, divided

1 small red onion, chopped

1 teaspoon dill

2 tablespoons nonfat plain yogurt

1 teaspoon mustard (preferably Dijon)

Salt and pepper to taste

Finely chop mushroom stems, leaving caps whole. Over high heat combine 1 tablespoon lemon juice with 1 quart water. Bring to a boil. Add mushroom caps and cook until tender. Transfer to a bowl filled with ice water. Drain and pat dry. In a separate bowl, combine red onion, dill, yogurt, mustard, and remaining lemon juice. Evenly divide filling among mushroom caps.

Salsa Dip

60 calories per serving

Makes 24 servings

1 pound processed cheese spread

1 eight ounce jar salsa

Microwave cheese spread and salsa in a two quart microwave safe bowl. Heat for 5 minutes on high. Stir after 3 minutes. Serve with baked tortilla chips, pepper wedges, or baked potato skins.

Pizza Potato Skins

65 calories per serving

Makes 24 servings

6 large baking potatoes

1 tablespoon oil

259

2 green peppers, diced

1 large onion, diced

2 ounce stick pepperoni, diced

1/4 teaspoon salt

1/4 teaspoon pepper

2 cans (8 ounces each) tomato sauce

2 tablespoons balsamic vinegar

2 ounces part skim shredded mozzarella cheese

Preheat oven to 400 degrees. Bake potatoes until tender. In a skillet, heat oil and add peppers, onion, pepperoni, salt, and pepper. Cook until vegetables are soft. Stir in sauce and vinegar. Cook until thickened and set aside. Cut potatoes lengthwise and scoop out potato, leaving shell. Cut lengthwise again. Transfer to baking sheet. Divide sauce evenly over potato strips. Sprinkle each with cheese. Bake until cheese is melted and skins are crisp.

Portobello-Stuffed Zucchini Boats

26 calories per serving

Makes 6 servings

3 medium zucchini, cut in half lengthwise

Olive oil nonstick cooking spray

2 portobello mushrooms, finely chopped

1 medium red pepper, finely chopped

1 tablespoon vinegar

3 tablespoons white wine

Preheat oven to 450 degrees. Scoop out insides of zucchini. Chop zucchini meat and set aside. Spray zucchini skins with oil and bake 10 minutes. Meanwhile, cook mushroom, pepper, zucchini meat, and vinegar in skillet over high heat. Add wine and cook until liquid is absorbed. Divide mixture among zucchini skins. Bake until tops are slightly browned.

Southwestern Popcorn Mix

75 calories per serving

Makes 8 servings

6 cups air popped popcorn

2 cups Cheerios cereal

2 tablespoons margarine

1/2 cup chili powder

1/2 cup garlic powder

2 tablespoons grated Parmesan cheese

Mix popcorn and cereal in large bowl. Heat margarine with chili and garlic powder until melted. Drizzle over mixture and toss until evenly coated. Sprinkle with cheese.

Black Bean and Corn Won Ton Cups

50 calories per serving

Makes 36 servings

36 won ton skins

1 cup chunky salsa

1 can whole kernel corn

1 can black beans, rinsed and drained

1/2 cup fat-free sour cream

Heat oven to 375 degrees. Line nonstick small muffin tins with won ton skins. Bake 10 minutes until golden. Remove from pan and cool. Mix remaining ingredients except sour cream. Spoon mixture evenly into cups. Top each with sour cream.

Appetizers
and Dips

Hot Spinach Dip

55 calories per serving

Makes 20 servings

1 8-ounce package cream cheese

1 cup fat-free sour cream

2 tablespoons lemon juice

2 tablespoons Worcestershire sauce

2 tablespoons milk

1 teaspoon mustard powder

2 packages (10 ounces) frozen chopped spinach, thawed and drained

1/2 cup diced red peppers

Preheat oven to 375 degrees. Beat together cream cheese, sour cream, lemon juice, Worcestershire, milk, and mustard powder until smooth. Gently stir in spinach and peppers. Bake in casserole dish until mixture bubbles around the edges. Serve with cut carrots, celery, etc.

Creamy Leek Dip

65 calories per serving

Makes 10 servings

2 cups low fat small curd cottage cheese

1/4 cup skim milk

1 packet leek soup mix

1 cup fresh parsley sprigs

In a food processor fitted with its metal blade, combine all ingredients except parsley sprigs until smooth. Add parsley and process until it is finely chopped. Place in a medium bowl and refrigerate for at least 2 hours.

Baked Onion Rings

51 calories per serving

Makes 4 servings

6 tablespoons seasoned dry bread crumbs

1/2 large sweet yellow onion

1 egg white

Preheat oven to 450 degrees. Slice onion as thinly as possible. Separate into rings. Dip onion first in egg white, then in bread crumbs. Place on a non-stick baking sheet. Bake 10 minutes.

Crab Meat Spread

28 calories per serving

Makes 12 servings

1 cup crab meat

1/2 cup celery, diced

1 small onion, diced

1/2 green pepper, diced

1 cup sprouts

1 cup low fat cottage cheese

Vinegar

Blend all above ingredients using enough vinegar to moisten. Season to taste.

Ham and Cheddar Bites

80 calories per serving
Makes 20 Servings

1 package (10 biscuits) refrigerated biscuit dough

3 tablespoons orange marmalade

1/4 cup water

1 tablespoon orange juice

1 teaspoon apple cider vinegar

1/2 teaspoon cumin

4 ounces sliced ham cut into 20 pieces

2 ounces cheddar cheese sliced into 20 pieces

Preheat oven to 350 degrees. Cut each biscuit dough piece in half crosswise and place on a baking sheet. Bake 10 minutes or until golden. Heat water and marmalade in small pan. Add orange juice, vinegar, and cumin. Cook until mixture thickens. Assemble by topping each biscuit with ham and cheese. Then top with marmalade mix.

Soups under 200 Calories

Chili Soup

175 calories per serving
Makes 5 servings

1/2 pound lean ground beef
1 tablespoon instant minced onion flakes
1 large can (16 ounces) red kidney beans, undrained
1 can (11 ounces) condensed reduced-fat tomato soup
1 soup can water
3 teaspoons chili powder

In a large pan, cook beef and onion over high heat until browned. Drain. Stir in remaining ingredients. Heat to boiling, stirring occasionally.

Egg Drop Soup

42 calories per serving
Makes 4 servings

2 cans (15 ounces) reduced-fat chicken stock
3 egg whites, slightly beaten
1 teaspoon soy sauce
1/4 cup chopped scallions

In a medium saucepan, bring chicken stock to a boil. Cook uncovered for 5 minutes to reduce volume. Add egg whites and cook, stirring occasionally until white and stringy. Remove from heat and stir in soy sauce and scallions.

265

Gazpacho

52 calories per serving

Makes 6 servings

1 cucumber, peeled, cut, and seeded

2 1/2 cups fresh tomatoes

1 large green pepper, chopped

1 large onion, chopped

1 teaspoon garlic flavoring

1 teaspoon dried chive

1 teaspoon paprika

Salt and pepper to taste

1/2 teaspoon sugar

2 cups tomato juice

2 tablespoons lemon juice

Shred cucumber with grater. Combine tomatoes, pepper, onion, garlic, chive, paprika, salt, and pepper. Add shredded cucumber to mixture. Stir in remaining ingredients. Cover and chill at least 2 hours before serving.

Yellow Pepper and Orange Soup

35 calories per serving

Makes 4 servings

2 yellow bell peppers, halved and seeded

1 large onion, chopped

Grated rind and juice of 1 orange

1 1/2 cups chicken stock

4 black olives, chopped

Salt and pepper to taste

Preheat oven to broil. Place peppers skin side up on baking sheet. Broil until skins are blackened. Cover and leave to cool. Place onion and orange juice in a small pan. Bring to a boil, then cover and simmer 10 minutes. Peel peppers and blend with onion, half of the orange rind, and chicken stock. Season to taste, then heat gently. Serve sprinkled with olives and remaining rind.

Vichyssoise

149 calories per serving
Makes 6 servings

3 medium leeks
3 potatoes, peeled and diced
3 cups chicken broth
2 cups evaporated skim milk
Freshly ground pepper

Cut and discard roots and tough leaves from leeks. Cut leeks in half lengthwise and rinse under cold water. Then cut leeks crosswise, into 1/4-inch thick slices.

Spray a saucepan with cooking spray. Heat the pan over medium heat. Add leeks, potatoes, and broth, cooking and stirring for 5 minutes. Reduce heat and simmer 30 minutes. Transfer leek mixture to food processor. Blend until smooth. Stir in milk and pepper. Soup may be chilled before serving.

Tortellini Soup

105 calories per serving
Makes 4 servings

3 cups beef broth
1 cup frozen cheese tortellini
1 cup frozen peas
2 tablespoons sun-dried tomatoes
1 teaspoon dried basil

In a medium saucepan, combine all ingredients. Cover and bring to a boil. Reduce heat and simmer 5 minutes or until tortellini are tender.

Vegetable Soup

75 calories per serving
Makes 8 servings

16 ounces tomato juice
16 ounces water
14 ounces chicken broth
16 ounces peeled tomatoes
1/2 pound green beans, cut into 1-inch pieces
3/4 pound carrots, sliced
3 celery stalks, sliced
1 onion, sliced
1 zucchini, sliced
1 summer squash, sliced

Combine tomato juice, water, broth, and tomatoes. Bring to a boil. Add remaining ingredients. Bring to a boil and simmer 30 minutes. Season to taste.

Mixed Bean Soup

95 calories a serving
Makes 4 servings

1 teaspoon olive oil
1 red onion, chopped
1 garlic clove, crushed
2/3 cup tomato paste
1 teaspoon dried thyme
1 1/2 cups frozen or fresh green beans
15-ounce can cannelloni beans
Salt and pepper to taste

Heat the olive oil in a pan, then sauté onion and garlic until tender but not brown. Add the tomato paste and thyme and bring to a boil. Add the green beans, cover and simmer for about 6 minutes or until tender. Add beans and season to taste.

Salads under 200 Calories

One Minute Chicken Salad

160 calories per serving

Makes 1 serving

5-ounce can premium chicken breast in water

2 tablespoons light mayonnaise

1 cup celery, diced

1 tablespoon finely diced onion

Drain chicken. Mix with mayonnaise, celery, and onion.

Greek Salad

90 calories per serving

Makes 2 servings

2 cups romaine lettuce

2 tablespoons feta cheese

1 tomato

1 cucumber

1/2 stalk celery, sliced

2 black olives

2 tablespoons vinegar

1 tablespoon olive oil

Toss all ingredients together and serve.

Salads

Fresh Pea Salad

70 calories per serving

Makes 12 servings

4 cups fresh peas

3 tablespoons fresh chive, chopped

2 tablespoons wine vinegar

2 tablespoons olive oil

1/2 teaspoon salt

2 red peppers, chopped

1 head Boston lettuce, thinly sliced

Over medium heat, bring peas and enough salted water to cover to a boil. Cook until tender. Rinse under cold water and drain. Whisk together chive, vinegar, oil, and salt. Add peas, peppers, and lettuce. Toss well to coat.

Citrus Salad

160 calories per serving

Makes 4 servings

2 seedless oranges

1 grapefruit

1 tablespoon honey

1 tablespoon olive oil

1 tablespoon balsamic vinegar

6 cups torn mixed greens

1 small red onion, sliced

Salt and pepper to taste

Peel oranges and grapefruit. Cut into 1/4-inch slices, then quarters. Combine olive oil, honey, and vinegar. Toss greens with dressing and red onion. Add orange and grapefruit pieces.

Noodle Salad

120 calories per serving

Makes 6 servings

8 ounces thin spaghetti

1 red pepper, sliced into thin strips

1 small cucumber, cut into thin strips

1/2 cup carrot, grated

2 green onions, thinly sliced

2 tablespoons rice vinegar

2 tablespoons teriyaki

2 tablespoons water

1 tablespoon soy sauce

1 teaspoon sesame oil

Cook spaghetti until just tender. Drain and rinse in cold water and transfer to large bowl. Add red pepper, cucumber, carrot, and onions, and mix well. In a small bowl, mix vinegar, teriyaki, water, soy sauce, and sesame oil. Pour sauce over noodle mix.

German Potato Salad

180 calories per serving

Makes 4 servings

1 1/2 pounds small red potatoes

3 shallots or leeks, minced

1/4 cup each of parsley, chive, and thyme

2 tablespoons balsamic or wine vinegar

2 tablespoons beef broth

2 tablespoons olive oil

2 garlic cloves, minced

Boil potatoes in saucepan until tender. Remove from heat, drain, and cut in halves. In a medium bowl, toss with shallots or leeks. Toss in parsley, chive, and thyme and set aside. In a small saucepan, combine vinegar, beef broth, olive oil, and garlic. Warm over low heat and pour over potatoes. Fold in carefully before serving.

271

Red Cole Slaw

40 calories per serving
Makes 4 servings

1/2 small red cabbage, shredded
1 red onion, thinly sliced
4 radishes, thinly sliced
1 red apple, cored and grated
1 tablespoon low fat plain yogurt
1 teaspoon honey
Salt and pepper to taste

Place cabbage, onion, radishes, and apple in salad bowl. Toss. In a screw top jar, shake the yogurt, honey, salt, and pepper until they are blended. Pour the dressing over the salad. Toss and serve.

Couscous Salad

105 calories per serving
Makes 4 servings

1 1/2 cups couscous
1 celery stalk, chopped
1/2 small cauliflower, cut into small florets
4 scallions, chopped
3 tablespoons dried parsley
1 tablespoon lemon juice
1/2 teaspoon chili sauce
Salt and pepper to taste

Cook couscous according to package directions. Leave to cool. Stir in remaining ingredients. Season and toss. Spoon onto a large platter and serve.

272

Deli Salad

180 calories per serving

Makes 8 servings

7-ounce can of artichoke hearts, drained

1 cup cubed mozzarella cheese

1 cup rotini pasta, cooked and drained

2 1/2-ounce cans pitted olives

1/2 cup low fat Italian dressing

1 cup red onion rings

1/2 cup green pepper, chopped

1/4 cup Parmesan cheese, shredded

Mix all ingredients together. Refrigerate before serving.

Spinach Salad

80 calories per serving

Makes 4 servings

2 cups fresh spinach

1/2 cup dried apricots, chopped

2 tablespoons sunflower seeds

1 tablespoon sesame seeds

2 tablespoons orange juice

1 tablespoon balsamic vinegar

2 tablespoons low fat plain yogurt

Salt and pepper to taste

Tear up spinach and place in large bowl. Add apricots, sunflower seeds, and sesame seeds. In a small bowl, mix together orange juice, vinegar, and yogurt. Pour over spinach mixture. Add salt and pepper. Refrigerate before serving.

Waldorf Salad

60 calories per serving
Makes 10 servings

6 cups apples, diced
2 1/2 cups celery, thinly sliced
1/2 cup raisins
1/2 cup nonfat mayonnaise
1/4 cup nonfat sour cream

Combine apples, celery, and raisins in a large bowl. Stir to mix well. In a small bowl, combine mayonnaise with sour cream. Stir. Add mayonnaise mixture to apple mixture and toss together. Refrigerate for 2 hours before serving.

Chicken and Pasta Salad

165 calories per serving
Makes 8 servings

3 cups chicken broth
1 pound boneless chicken breasts
2 cups shell pasta
1 cup nonfat mayonnaise
1 teaspoon mustard
1/2 teaspoon celery salt
Ground pepper to taste
2 ribs of celery, thinly sliced
1 cup baby peas, cooked, drained, and cooled
1 cup seedless red grapes, washed and cut in half

Bring chicken broth to a simmer in medium saucepan. Add chicken breasts and cook for 20 minutes. Remove breasts and chill. Cook pasta according to directions, drain, and rinse in cold water. Mix together mayonnaise, mustard, celery salt, and pepper. Cut chicken into bite-size pieces and add to mixture. Add pasta, celery, peas, and grapes. Toss together. Cover and refrigerate one hour.

Arugula and Orange Salad

50 calories per serving

Makes 6 servings

1 bunch arugula, stems removed

9 radishes, thinly sliced

1 red onion, thinly sliced

1 orange, peeled and sectioned

1 tablespoon chicken broth

Juice and grated zest of 1 lime

1 clove garlic, minced

1/2 teaspoon ground cumin

1/2 teaspoon salt

1 teaspoon olive oil

Combine arugula, radishes, onion, and orange sections. In separate bowl combine chicken broth, lime juice and zest, garlic, cumin, and salt. Whisk in oil until mixture thickens slightly. Add to salad.

Cucumber Salad with Dill

50 calories per serving

Makes 4 servings

2 cucumbers

3 tablespoons vinegar

1 tablespoon sugar

Salt and pepper to taste

1 red onion, sliced and made into rings

1 teaspoon dried dill weed

Wash the cucumbers and partially remove peel in lengthwise strips. Use a fork to leave a little skin between each strip and slice crosswise. Combine

Salads

275

vinegar, sugar, salt, and pepper in a bowl until sugar is dissolved. Add cucumber, onion, and dill. Toss well. Serve immediately.

Vegetable Salad

55 calories per serving
Makes 8 servings

3 cups broccoli, chopped
3 cups cauliflower, chopped
1 cup celery, sliced
20 black olives, pitted and sliced
15-ounce can mushrooms, drained
3/4 cup fat-free Italian salad dressing

Combine all ingredients in a large bowl. Stir to cover vegetables. Chill at least 3 hours before serving.

Low Fat Salad Dressings

Creamy Ranch Dressing

15 calories per tablespoon
Makes 1 cup

3/4 cup plain nonfat yogurt
1/4 cup low fat mayonnaise
1 tablespoon cider vinegar
2 teaspoons Dijon mustard
1/4 teaspoon dried thyme
1 green onion, minced

Mix all ingredients together. Cover and refrigerate.
Stir before serving.

Creamy Italian Dressing

10 calories per tablespoon
Makes 1 cup

1/2 cup fat-free sour cream
1/3 cup nonfat buttermilk
2 tablespoons grated Parmesan cheese
1 teaspoon dried basil, crushed
1 clove garlic, minced
Salt and pepper to taste

Mix the sour cream and buttermilk in a small bowl
until smooth. Stir in Parmesan, basil, garlic, salt,
and pepper. Refrigerate.

277

Vegetable Dishes under 200 Calories

Snow Peas and Carrots

80 calories per serving
Makes 4 servings

1 onion, thinly sliced
4 teaspoons olive oil
2 carrots, cut into 2-inch strips
1/2 pound snow peas, strings removed
2 teaspoons dried dill
Salt and pepper to taste

Microwave onion and oil for 1 minute. Stir in carrots, cover with plastic, and microwave for 2 minutes. Stir in snow peas and dill. Microwave covered for 6 minutes. Let stand for 3 minutes. Season and serve.

Carrots and Grapes

45 calories per serving
Makes 4 servings

2 cups carrots, sliced
1 shallot, chopped
1/4 cup water
2 tablespoons red wine vinegar
1 tablespoon brown sugar
1/2 cup seedless grapes, halved

In nonstick skillet, cook carrots and shallot in water for about 10 minutes. Stir until carrots are tender. Push carrot mixture to side of skillet. Stir in vinegar and sugar. Gently add in grapes. Toss all together.

Hash Browns

96 calories per serving

Makes 4 servings

4 medium-size potatoes
1 onion
Nonfat cooking spray
Paprika

Preheat oven to 400 degrees. Cut potatoes into cubes. Cut onion into small pieces. Spray 9 x 9-inch pan with cooking spray. Place cut potatoes and onion in pan. Sprinkle with a little water, then sprinkle with paprika. Bake for 20 minutes, then remove from oven. Heat oven to broiling, then cook mixture until potatoes are brown.

Zucchini Frittata

65 calories per serving

Makes 4 servings

2 small zucchini
1 teaspoon water
2 green onions, chopped
1 teaspoon basil
1 teaspoon dried marjoram
1 1/2 cups egg substitute
2 tablespoons Parmesan cheese

Cut each zucchini lengthwise into quarters. Thinly slice each quarter. Place the water in a 10-inch skillet. Add zucchini and onions. Cook over low heat about 3 minutes. Discard cooking liquid. Stir in basil and marjoram. Carefully pour egg substitute over zucchini and onions. Cook over low heat until mixture starts to set. Lift edges of uncooked

Vegetable Dishes

279

mixture to flow underneath. Continue cooking until nearly set. Sprinkle with cheese. Broil 1 minute and serve.

Peas and Onions

105 calories per serving

Makes 8 servings

16-ounce package frozen small whole onions

2 tablespoons butter

20 ounces frozen peas, thawed

2 tablespoons chopped mint

1 tablespoon Parmesan cheese

Salt and pepper to taste

Cook onions according to package directions. Drain. Melt butter in skillet and add onions and peas cooking for 3 minutes. Place in bowl, toss with mint, cheese, salt, and pepper.

Rosemary "Fries"

75 calories per serving

Makes 4 servings

3 large baking potatoes

2 teaspoons olive oil

1 teaspoon rosemary

Salt and pepper to taste

Preheat broiler. Cut potatoes lengthwise into 3 slices each. Cut each slice into 3 large French fries. Cook potatoes in microwave with a bit of water. Take out while still crisp (not mashing soft). Spread steamed potatoes on baking sheet sprayed with cooking spray. Sprinkle with olive oil and dried rosemary. Broil until potatoes are golden brown. Turn and brown other side. Season and serve.

Vegetable Dishes

Sesame Broccoli and Cauliflower

50 calories per serving

Makes 1 serving

1/4 cup cauliflower florets

3/4 cup broccoli

1/2 teaspoon soy sauce

1/4 teaspoon sesame oil

Salt and pepper to taste

Combine soy sauce, sesame oil, salt, and pepper in microwave-proof bowl. Add broccoli and cauliflower. Cover and microwave on high for 1 minute. Uncover and toss.

Orange-Glazed Asparagus

45 calories per serving

Makes 8 servings

2 tablespoons butter

2 packages (10 ounces each) frozen asparagus

1/4 cup orange juice

1/4 cup white wine

1 teaspoon orange peel

Salt and pepper to taste

In large skillet, melt butter over medium heat. Add asparagus and cook until heated through. Transfer to a dish. In same skillet, add orange juice, wine, peel, salt, and pepper. Cook until reduced by half. Pour over asparagus.

Vegetable Dishes

281

Glazed Carrots

70 calories per serving

Makes 4 servings

1 pound carrots
1 cup water
4 teaspoons apple juice
1 tablespoon brown sugar
1 teaspoon butter
1/2 teaspoon nutmeg

Cut carrots into 2-inch pieces, then quarter them lengthwise. Microwave carrots for 5 minutes until just tender. Meanwhile, stir together water, apple juice, brown sugar, and butter. Microwave for 30 seconds or until sugar and butter just melt. Drizzle carrots with juice mixture. Toss to coat. Serve sprinkled with nutmeg.

Rice Almondine

115 calories per serving

Makes 6 servings

1 cup onion, chopped
1 1/4 cups chicken broth
1 tablespoon lemon juice
1/2 teaspoon garlic powder
1 1/2 cups minute brown rice
1 cup frozen green beans, thawed
2 tablespoons toasted slivered almonds
1/2 teaspoon dried dill weed.

Coat medium saucepan with cooking spray. Add onion and cook until tender. Add chicken broth, lemon juice, and garlic powder. Bring to a boil. Stir in rice and return to a boil. Reduce heat to low. Cover and simmer about 5 minutes. Remove from heat and stir in remaining ingredients. Fluff with fork and serve.

Swiss Asparagus Au Gratin

170 calories per serving

Makes 4 servings

1/2 cup water

1 1/2 pounds asparagus spears, trimmed

1/2 cup Swiss cheese, shredded

1/4 cup bread crumbs

2 tablespoons butter, melted

1/2 teaspoon dry mustard

1/4 teaspoon fresh ground pepper

Heat oven to 400 degrees. Bring 1/2 cup water to a boil in 10-inch skillet. Add asparagus. Cook 2 minutes and drain. Place in 10 x 6-inch baking pan. Mix remaining ingredients. Sprinkle over asparagus. Bake 10 minutes until cheese mixture is lightly browned.

Vegetable Dishes

Entrees under 200 Calories

Beef Tenderloin with Onions

175 calories per serving

Makes 4 servings

1/2 cup chicken broth

2 large onions, thinly sliced

4 cloves garlic, finely chopped

1/4 cup balsamic vinegar

1/2 teaspoon salt

1/4 teaspoon ground pepper

4 beef tenderloin steaks (totalling 1 pound)

Heat chicken broth to boiling in a 1-quart saucepan. Stir in onions and garlic. Cover and

cook over medium heat until onions are soft. Stir in vinegar and cook uncovered until liquid has evaporated. Sprinkle beef with salt and pepper. Cook beef in nonstick skillet until desired doneness. Serve with onions.

Broiled Flank Steak

170 calories per serving

Makes 4 servings

1 pound lean flank steak

3/4 cup dry red wine

3 garlic cloves, cut into quarters

1 bay leaf, cut in half

1 teaspoon onion powder

2 teaspoons Dijon mustard

Marinate steak in a baking dish with wine, garlic,

and bay leaf for 1 hour. Preheat broiler. Drain steak. Place steak on a broiler rack. Sprinkle with onion powder. Spread a thin layer of mustard over the top. Broil to desired doneness.

Combine soy sauce, water, garlic powder, and apple sauce. Marinate over steak 1 hour. Thread steak, pepper, pineapple, and mushrooms on skewers. Broil until desired doneness.

Pineapple Steak Kabobs

185 calories per serving
Makes 4 servings

1 tablespoon soy sauce
2 tablespoons water
1 teaspoon garlic powder
1 tablespoon apple sauce
1 pound steak, cut into 2-inch squares
Small red bell pepper, cut into 1-inch squares
8-ounce can unsweetened pineapple chunks, juice reserved
8 fresh mushrooms

Meat Loaf

150 calories per serving
Makes 4 servings

3/4 pound lean ground beef
3/4 pound ground turkey breast
1/2 cup old-fashioned oatmeal
1/2 cup tomato puree
1 teaspoon Italian seasoning
1/2 teaspoon salt
1 small onion, chopped
1 clove garlic, finely chopped

Preheat oven to 375 degrees. Mix all ingredients

Entrees

285

thoroughly. Press mixture into ungreased loaf pan. Bake about one hour or until center is no longer pink.

Pork Steaks with Peppercorn Glaze

175 calories per serving
Makes 4 servings

4 lean pork loin steaks
1 tablespoon green peppercorns, crushed
4 tablespoons balsamic vinegar
1/2 cup chicken broth
4 scallions, sliced

Mix together peppercorns and vinegar. Sprinkle over pork. Marinate for 30 minutes. Reserving the peppercorn mixture, fry the pork in a nonstick pan. Add the peppercorn mix, broth, and scallions. Boil rapidly, uncovered, for about 10 minutes.

Lemon Chicken

130 calories per serving
Makes 4 servings

1 pound boneless chicken breast halves (4 pieces)
2 lemons
1 teaspoon dried tarragon
Fresh pepper to taste

Preheat oven to 350 degrees. Place chicken in foil-lined baking pan. Fold sides of the foil up. Halve lemons and squeeze juice of 1/2 lemon over each chicken piece. Sprinkle each piece with 1/4 teaspoon tarragon and pepper to taste. Fold foil together and seal to secure chicken. Bake for about 45 minutes.

Feta and Mint Chicken Breasts

160 calories per serving

Makes 4 servings

4 6-ounce boneless, skinless chicken breast halves

1 ounce feta cheese, thinly sliced

1 cup fresh mint leaves

2 teaspoons olive oil

1 tablespoon lemon juice

Salt and pepper to taste

Pressing each breast, cut a pocket. Insert feta cheese and half of mint leaves evenly into each breast. Place breasts in baking dish. Finely chop remaining mint and add olive oil, lemon juice, salt, and pepper. Marinate for 30 minutes. Preheat broiler. Broil 4 to 6 minutes per side.

Mediterranean Turkey Spirals

125 calories per serving

Makes 4 servings

4 thin turkey breast steaks

2 tablespoons pesto

1/2 cup basil leaves

1/2 cup chicken broth

1/2 cup tomato juice

Garlic, salt, and pepper to taste

Pound turkey until thin. Spread with pesto sauce. Lay basil leaves over each steak, then roll in a jelly roll fashion. Secure with toothpicks. Combine chicken broth and tomato juice. Bring to a boil over high heat. Add the turkey spirals, cover, and simmer for 15 minutes. Season, and remove toothpicks. Serve hot.

Entrees

287

Entrees

Turkey Meat Loaf

175 calories per serving

Makes 8 servings

1 1/2 pounds ground turkey breast

1/2 cup seasoned bread crumbs

1/2 cup uncooked oatmeal

1/2 cup low fat milk

2 tablespoons soy sauce

1 large onion, chopped

1 egg

Fresh ground pepper

Preheat oven to 350 degrees. Mix all ingredients. Place mixture in a loaf pan coated with cooking spray. Bake about 1 hour. Meat should not have any pink color when done.

Tuna with Tomato Vinaigrette

110 calories per serving

Makes 6 servings

1 1/2 cup water

1/2 cup sun-dried tomatoes

2 cloves garlic, sliced

1/4 cup olive oil

1/4 cup lemon juice

1 tablespoon dried thyme

6 tuna steaks (about 6 ounces each)

Salt and pepper to taste

Preheat broiler. Over medium heat, bring 1 1/2 cups water to a boil. Add sun-dried tomatoes and cook until softened. Drain and reserve liquid. Cook garlic in olive oil until golden. Stir in tomatoes, lemon juice, thyme, and reserved liquid and leave simmering. Separately, sprinkle tuna with salt and pepper and broil until done. Top with simmering sauce.

Baked Scallops

125 calories per serving

Makes 4 servings

1 tablespoon butter

1/4 cup white wine

Juice from one lemon

1 pound scallops

Preheat oven to 450 degrees. Heat all but the scallops in oven for 10 minutes. Pour liquid over scallops. Marinate in 9-inch casserole pan for 20 minutes at room temperature. Bake for about 15 minutes. Do not overcook.

Oysters Rockefeller

90 calories per serving

Makes 4 servings

2 teaspoons olive oil

1 tablespoon onion, grated

2 tablespoons bread crumbs

Tarragon, pepper, and Tabasco to taste

10 ounces frozen chopped spinach, thawed and drained

8 ounces oysters, raw or canned

2 tablespoons mozzarella cheese, grated

1 tablespoon Parmesan cheese

Preheat broiler. Combine oil, onion, bread crumbs, and seasoning. Toss mixture with spinach. Broil oysters for 5 to 7 minutes if using raw oysters. Drain liquid if using canned oysters. Top oysters with spinach mixture and broil about 4 minutes. Sprinkle with cheeses and broil until just melted.

Entrees

Deviled Shrimp

140 calories per serving

Makes 1 serving

5 jumbo shrimp, uncooked, peeled, and deveined
2 tablespoons white wine
1 tablespoon Dijon mustard
1 garlic clove, crushed
1/4 cup onions, diced
Salt and pepper to taste
1 tomato, peeled
1/4 cup parsley, chopped

Coat skillet with cooking spray. Add shrimp and cook on high heat about 2 minutes on each side. Add wine, mustard, garlic, onion, and seasonings. Cover and cook about 8 minutes. Add tomato, breaking it up with a fork. Mix all together, cover again, and cook 10 minutes. Add parsley and serve.

Seafood Bisque

130 calories per serving

Makes 8 servings

2 1/2 cups frozen corn, thawed
2 cups chicken broth
1 tablespoon butter
2 green peppers, chopped
Salt and pepper to taste
1 cup low fat milk
1/2 pound shrimp, peeled and deveined
1/2 pound scallops
3 tablespoons parsley

In food processor, combine 2 cups corn with 1 cup chicken broth. Purée until smooth. Melt butter over medium heat in a saucepan. Add peppers, onions, salt, and pepper to taste. Cook 5 minutes. Stir in corn mixture, milk, and remaining broth. Cover and simmer 5 minutes. Add shrimp, scallops, remaining corn, and parsley. Cook about 5 minutes and serve.

Entrees

Stir-Fried Tofu with Vegetables

150 calories per serving
Makes 4 servings

2 teaspoons vegetable oil
1 package (16 ounces) extra firm tofu, patted dry
and cut into 1-inch pieces
1 cup vegetable broth
1 tablespoon soy sauce
2 teaspoons flour
3 green onions, thinly sliced
1 bag (10 ounces) shredded carrots
1 medium red pepper, thinly sliced
2 garlic cloves, crushed in garlic press
1 tablespoon ginger
1/2 teaspoon salt

In a skillet, heat 1 teaspoon vegetable oil until hot, then add tofu. Cook 4 minutes until golden. Transfer to plate and set aside. In a separate bowl, mix vegetable broth, soy sauce, and flour. In the same skillet, heat remaining teaspoon oil, white parts of green onions, carrots, pepper, garlic, ginger, and salt. Cook 5 minutes, stirring frequently. Return tofu to skillet and stir in broth mixture. Heat to boiling and serve.

Baked Eggplant, Tomatoes, and Feta

95 calories per serving
Makes 4 servings

1 medium eggplant, thinly sliced
Garlic salt to taste
2 large tomatoes, sliced
1 cup feta cheese, crumbled

Entrees

291

4 tablespoons plain yogurt

Paprika to taste

Preheat oven to 400 degrees. Sprinkle the eggplant slices with garlic salt, leave for 30 minutes, then wipe salt off. Spray baking dish with cooking spray. Arrange eggplant and tomatoes to slightly overlap. Sprinkle with feta cheese and spoon over yogurt. Sprinkle with paprika and garlic salt. Bake for 30 minutes or until bubbling and golden.

Vegetable Tortillas

180 calories per serving

Makes 6 servings

1/2 cup red pepper, diced

1/2 cup yellow pepper, diced

1/2 cup zucchini, diced

6 flour tortillas

1 1/2 cups reduced-fat Monterey Jack cheese, shredded

Mix peppers and zucchini. Spoon 1/4 cup of vegetable mixture onto center of each tortilla. Top each with 1/4 cup cheese. Roll tortilla tightly around mixture. Spray 10-inch skillet with non-stick cooking spray. Cook 3 tortillas seam side down until bottoms are light brown. Spray tops and turn. Cook 3 minutes longer until brown. Repeat with remaining tortillas.

Entrees

292

Enchiladas

160 calories per serving

Makes 6 servings

2 cups chunky salsa

Vegetable cooking spray

1 red bell pepper, thinly sliced

1/2 cup onion, thinly sliced

2 cups mushrooms, sliced

1 small potato, cut into 1/2-inch pieces

1 clove garlic, minced

1/4 cup water

2 cups fresh spinach leaves, washed and dried

1/4 teaspoon hot red pepper flakes

1/2 cup feta cheese, crumbled

6 corn tortillas

8 cups Romaine lettuce, finely shredded

Preheat oven to 375 degrees. Lightly spray 10-inch nonstick skillet with cooking spray. Add pepper and onion and cook until softened. Add mushrooms, potato, garlic, and 1/4 cup water and cook until softened. Remove from heat and stir in spinach and pepper flakes until spinach is wilted. Add feta and stir to blend. Warm tortillas in skillet, about a minute each side. Place 1/3 cup of vegetable mixture in tortilla and roll up. Lightly spray square baking pan and place tortillas seam side down. Brush lightly with a little liquid from salsa. Cover with foil and bake for 20 minutes. Divide lettuce among 6 plates and place enchiladas on top. Top with salsa.

Entrees

Vegetarian Stuffed Peppers

145 calories per serving

Makes 6 servings

6 green peppers

2 cups cooked rice

1 cup couscous

3 egg whites

Salt, pepper, and parsley to taste

1/4 cup seasoned bread crumbs

1 cup water

1 small onion, chopped

1/2 cup celery, chopped

8-ounce can tomato sauce

Preheat oven to 375 degrees. Cut peppers in half and remove seeds. Microwave 2 minutes. Combine rice, cooked couscous, egg whites, and seasonings. Sprinkle in bread crumbs and set aside as stuffing. Bring 1 cup water to a boil. Add onion and celery, boil 15 more minutes. Add tomato sauce, mix, and cook 20 minutes. Spray a baking dish with cooking spray. Fill peppers with stuffing. Cover with sauce. Bake for 40 minutes.

Entrees

Pasta Primavera

180 calories per serving

Makes 4 servings

8 ounces uncooked linguine

1 cup green beans, in 1-inch pieces

1 medium carrot, cut into 1/4-inch slices

1/2 medium green pepper

1 cup mushrooms, sliced

1 medium tomato, cut into 1-inch pieces

8-ounce bottle fat-free creamy Italian dressing

Cook linguine until tender, adding green beans, carrot, and pepper during last 5 minutes. While linguine is cooking, place mushrooms in colander. Drain linguine and vegetables in colander. Place linguine mixture in saucepan, adding in tomato and dressing. Cook over medium heat until hot.

Entrees

Breads, Pizza, and Quiche under 200 Calories

Lemon Pepper Popovers

105 calories per serving
Makes 6 servings

1 cup flour
1 cup skim milk at room temperature
1 tablespoon olive oil
Salt and pepper to taste
2 teaspoons lemon zest
3 egg whites, slightly beaten

Preheat oven to 450 degrees. Mix together flour and milk. Add remaining ingredients, just enough to mix. Grease muffin cups with cooking spray.

Fill each cup half full. Bake 15 minutes at 450 degrees. Reduce heat to 350 degrees for 20 more minutes. Serve at once.

Blueberry Muffins

123 calories per serving
Makes 12 muffins

2 cups flour
1 tablespoon baking powder
1/2 teaspoon salt
1 cup blueberries
4 egg whites
1 1/2 cups nonfat yogurt
1/2 cup sugar
1 teaspoon vanilla extract

Preheat oven to 400 degrees. Mix together flour, baking powder, and salt. Add blueberries. Stir lightly to coat and set aside. Beat egg whites to peaks. Add yogurt, sugar, and vanilla. Add liquid mixture to dry ingredients and fold together gently. Place in nonstick 12-cup muffin pan. Optional: Place 1 blueberry in the center of each muffin. Sprinkle a little sugar over each muffin. Bake for 20 minutes.

Spiced Carrot Bread

125 calories per serving
Makes one loaf or 12 slices

2 eggs
4 tablespoons vegetable oil
3 tablespoons sugar
3 carrots, coarsely grated
1 1/3 cups flour
1 teaspoon baking powder
2 teaspoons allspice
3 tablespoons skim milk

Preheat oven to 350 degrees. Line loaf pan with wax paper. Mix together eggs, oil, and sugar. Stir in carrots. Add flour, baking powder, and allspice. Fold in milk. Pour into pan. Bake 40 to 45 minutes.

Pizza Bread

135 calories per serving
Makes 6 servings

1 1/2 cups flour
1 1/2 teaspoons baking powder
1/2 teaspoon salt
3/4 cup beer
1/2 cup spaghetti sauce
1/3 cup low fat mozzarella cheese, shredded

Heat oven to 400 degrees. Spray round cake pan with nonstick cooking spray. Mix flour, baking

Breads, Pizza, and Quiche

297

powder, and salt in mixing bowl. Thoroughly stir in beer. Spread dough in pan and spread sauce over it. Bake 15 minutes or until toothpick inserted in center comes out clean.

Spicy Onion Tart

175 calories per serving

Makes 8 servings

1 tablespoon butter

4 large yellow onions, thinly sliced

1 cup nonfat sour cream

3 eggs

Salt, black pepper, and cayenne pepper to taste

One frozen pie shell

1 teaspoon dried parsley

Preheat oven to 375 degrees. Melt butter in large nonstick skillet. Add onions. Cover and cook 15 minutes. Uncover and cook until browned. Remove from heat and let cool. Combine sour cream, eggs, peppers, and salt. Add onions. Pour into pie shell. Sprinkle with parsley. Bake 30 to 35 minutes. Cool slightly before slicing.

Breads, Pizza, and Quiche

298

Onion Twists

120 calories per serving
Makes 12 servings

1 large onion, thinly sliced
2 tablespoons olive oil
2 tablespoons parsley, minced
1/2 teaspoon coarse salt
1 pound frozen pizza dough, thawed
1 egg, beaten

Preheat oven to 400 degrees. Heat oil in skillet and cook onion over medium heat until golden. Stir in parsley and 1/4 teaspoon salt. Roll dough out on floured surface to about 15 x 12-inches. Spread onion on lower half of dough, leaving a border. Fold dough lengthwise, seal, and brush with egg. Cut crosswise into 12 strips. Twist and place on nonstick baking pan. Brush with egg and sprinkle with remaining egg and salt. Bake until golden.

Broiled Crisp Bread

100 calories per serving
Makes 12 servings

2 cups flour
1 teaspoon salt
4 tablespoons butter, melted
1/2 cup warm water
1 teaspoon red pepper flakes
Salt and pepper to taste

Preheat broiler. Combine flour and salt. Stir in 2 tablespoons butter. Stir in water 1 tablespoon at a time. Divide dough into 12 pieces and roll each piece into a circle. Coat baking pan with cooking spray. Broil circles for 2 minutes on each side, brushing with butter. Sprinkle with salt, pepper, and flakes. Broil one more minute.

Breads, Pizza, and Quiche

299

Desserts under 200 Calories

Lemon Bars

150 calories per serving

Makes 24 bars

1 cup shortening

1 cup brown sugar

1 1/2 cups flour

1 teaspoon baking powder

1 teaspoon cinnamon

1 cup quick cooking oats

8 ounces light cream cheese, softened

1/2 cup sugar

1/2 cup lemon juice

2 teaspoons grated lemon peel

Preheat oven to 350 degrees. Beat together shortening and brown sugar. Add flour, baking powder, and cinnamon. Stir in oats. Reserve $1^1/_2$ cups oat mixture. Press remaining oat mixture onto bottom of greased 13 x 9-inch pan. Beat cream cheese with sugar, juice, and peel. Pour over oat mixture. Sprinkle with remaining mixture. Bake about 30 minutes.

Desserts

Apple Crisp

135 calories per serving

Makes 8 servings

4 apples, sliced

1/3 cup brown sugar

1/4 cup flour

1/4 cup rolled oats

1 teaspoon cinnamon

2 tablespoons butter, softened

Preheat oven to 375 degrees. Coat an 8 x 8-inch pan with cooking spray. Place apple slices in pan. Mix remaining ingredients together. Sprinkle over apples. Bake 30 minutes.

Apple Nut Cookies

75 calories per serving

Makes 14 cookies

1 1/2 cups rolled oats

1 teaspoon allspice

4 tablespoons shortening

3 tablespoons brown sugar

1 apple, cored and chopped

3 tablespoons walnuts

1 egg white

Preheat oven to 400 degrees. Mix together oats, allspice, and shortening. Add brown sugar, apple, walnuts, and egg white. Stir. Form 14 balls. Arrange on nonstick baking pan. Flatten slightly. Bake for 10 minutes.

Desserts

Chocolate Truffles

60 calories per serving

Makes about 30 truffles

1/2 cup chopped raisins

2 tablespoons chocolate flavored liqueur

40 squares graham crackers ground to a powder

14-ounce can sweetened condensed skim milk

1/2 cup unsweetened cocoa powder

1 teaspoon vanilla

Combine raisins and liqueur. Let stand until softened. Combine crackers, milk, 1/4 cup cocoa powder, vanilla, and raisin mixture. Chill one hour. Place remaining cocoa powder in shallow bowl. Shape chocolate mixture into balls. Roll in cocoa powder. Freeze 15 minutes. Store in refrigerator.

Biscotti

65 calories per serving

Makes 24 servings

3 cups flour

1 teaspoon baking powder

5 tablespoons shortening

2/3 cup sugar

3 eggs

1 tablespoon lemon juice

1 cup currants

3/4 cup dried apricots

Preheat oven to 350 degrees. Combine flour and baking powder. Set aside. Cream together shortening and sugar. Beat in eggs. Add lemon juice. Add dry ingredients. Add currants and apricots. Divide and shape dough into 2 loaves. Bake 30 minutes.

Cheesecake Cups

129 calories per serving

Makes 8 servings

1 quart low fat yogurt

3 tablespoons sugar

1 teaspoon lemon juice

2 slices pumpernickel bread

2 tablespoons honey

1 cup mandarin orange sections

Strain yogurt and refrigerate 4 hours. Stir in lemon juice and sugar. Refrigerate another 4 hours. Preheat oven to 375 degrees. Toast bread, crumble, and add honey. Press into bottom of 8 cups to make crust. Cover with yogurt mixture. Add a couple of orange sections on top.

Chocolate Kisses

20 calories per serving

Makes 30 servings

3 tablespoons cocoa powder

1/2 cup confectioners' sugar

4 egg whites

1/2 teaspoon lemon juice

1/2 cup granulated sugar

Preheat oven to 250 degrees. Line a baking pan with waxed paper. Sift together cocoa powder and confectioners' sugar and set aside. Beat egg whites and lemon juice until soft peaks form. Add 1 1/2 tablespoons granulated sugar and beat until stiff. Add remaining sugar and beat again until glossy. Fold in cocoa mixture. Spoon into small "kiss" shapes on baking sheet. Bake for 2 hours, then turn off oven and let set 1 hour. Cool completely.

303

Desserts

Blueberry Cake

125 calories per serving

Makes 15 servings

1 cup frozen blueberries, thawed

1 1/2 tablespoons sugar

2 tablespoons margarine

2 tablespoons corn syrup

1/2 cup egg substitute

2 teaspoons almond extract

3 cups flour

1 1/4 teaspoons baking soda

1 1/4 cups nonfat sour cream

1/3 cup powdered sugar

2 teaspoons skim milk

Preheat oven to 375 degrees. Spray bundt pan with nonfat cooking spray. Blend blueberries and sugar until smooth, set aside. In a medium bowl, combine margarine, corn syrup, egg substitute, and 1 teaspoon almond extract. Add flour, baking soda, and sour cream. Combine 3/4 cup batter with blueberry mixture. Spread 2/3 of batter into pan, top with blueberry mix. Finish with remaining batter. Bake 40 minutes. Combine powdered sugar, 1 teaspoon almond extract, and skim milk. Drizzle over cooled cake.

Skim Milk Custard

90 calories per serving

Makes 4 servings

2 cups cold skim milk

1 tablespoon unflavored gelatin

3 tablespoons sugar

1 teaspoon almond extract

Pour milk into saucepan and sprinkle gelatin in. Let stand 5 minutes. Stir over low heat until gelatin is dissolved. Stir in sugar and cook for 3 minutes, stirring constantly. Remove from heat and stir in extract. Pour into 4 ramekins and chill until set.

S'mores Fudge

25 calories per serving

Makes 60 servings

8-ounce package reduced-fat chocolate baking chips

2/3 cup nonfat sweetened condensed milk

1 teaspoon vanilla extract

1 1/3 cups miniature marshmallows

2 low fat graham crackers, broken in small pieces

Line 8-inch baking pan with waxed paper. In nonstick saucepan, over low heat, stir chocolate chips and condensed milk until melted. Remove from heat and cool 2 minutes, then stir in vanilla extract and 1 cup marshmallows. Pour into pan, sticking graham cracker pieces and remaining marshmallows into fudge. Refrigerate until firm. Peel off waxed paper, invert, and cut into 1-inch squares.

305

Desserts

Sugar and Spice Doughnuts

125 calories per serving

Makes 10 servings

2 cups reduced-fat biscuit mix

3 tablespoons sugar

1/4 teaspoon nutmeg

1/2 cup buttermilk

1/4 cup egg substitute

1 tablespoon melted butter

1/4 teaspoon cinnamon

Preheat oven to 425 degrees. Combine biscuit mix, 1 tablespoon sugar, nutmeg, buttermilk, and egg substitute. Knead dough on floured surface for 10 strokes. Roll out to 1/2-inch thickness. Cut with doughnut cutter and bake for 10 minutes. Combine remaining sugar and cinnamon. Brush doughnuts with butter and dip into cinnamon/sugar mixture.

Fruit Skewers with Mango Purée

80 calories per serving

Makes 4 servings

1 ripe mango, peeled, pitted, and chopped

1 tablespoon lime juice

1/2 pineapple, cored

1 papaya, peeled and seeded

2 kiwi, peeled and quartered

Place mango and lime juice in a food processor and blend. Cut pineapple and papaya into bite-sized chunks and thread on skewer with kiwi. To serve, spoon a little mango purée on four plates. Place cooked skewer on top.

Molasses Cookies

50 calories per serving
Makes 40 cookies

1/2 cup light molasses
1/3 cup shortening
2 cups flour
1/4 cup brown sugar
1 tablespoon skim milk
1 teaspoon ginger
1/2 teaspoon baking powder

In a pan, heat molasses to boiling and stir in shortening until melted. Remove from heat and stir in flour, brown sugar, milk, ginger, and baking powder. Stir until mixture pulls away from pan. After dough cools, form into 1-inch thick log. Refrigerate until firm. Preheat oven to 350 degrees. Slice into 1/4-inch slices. Bake on non-stick cookie sheet for 10 minutes.

307

Desserts

A Final Word

Remember This!

Through the years of researching what works and what doesn't in the world of dieting, I found that each and every one of us must walk our own path. The biggest successes for the people I interviewed came only after they stopped trying to conform to someone else's philosophy of eating or living. When they finally decided that no one else on the planet could possibly know what they were feeling or needing, they could develop their own program and finally win their battle. The program that you choose has to be based on your lifestyle, schedule, likes, and dislikes. Best of luck in your pursuit of finding the program that works for you. You can do it. It takes creativity, patience, and all the willpower and courage you know you carry within.

About the Author

Being in front of an audience comes naturally to Diane Irons, who began her career as a model at age fourteen. She then moved on to become a highly successful journalist and internationally known fashion and image expert. Her consumer approach to beauty, diet, and cosmetics has helped thousands of women realize that glamour and style are every woman's birthright and should be inexpensive, simple, and fun. Diane has worked as a spokesperson for such companies as Hawaiian Tropic, Vogue/Butterick, Barbizon International, Simplicity, and Conde Naste.

Irons has also lent her expertise on the nation's top shows and the world's most prestigious publications, including *Good Morning America*, *Entertainment Tonight*, *Inside Edition*, *CNBC*, *Maury Povich*, *Montel Williams*, *CNN*, *The Gayle King Show*, *Crook & Chase*, *Wall Street Journal*, *Los Angeles Times*, *Chicago Tribune*, *Boston Globe*, *New York Post*, *National Examiner*, *Cosmopolitan* and *Self*.

The World's Best-Kept Diet Secrets is a follow-up to her *USA Today* bestseller, **The World's Best-Kept Beauty Secrets**. With her commitment to uncovering the hype and harm, Irons can be relied upon to bring accurate, cutting-edge news from inside the world of image. When it comes to the diet and beauty industry, she is a leading force in accurate consumer information.

Index

3rd Rock from the Sun, 93

A

A-1 General Vitamin, 214
Ab machine, 131
Acids, 232
Acupuncture, 30
Adipose tissue, 115
Adrenal cortex extract, 35
Age spot, 125
Aging, 94, 161
Air conditioning, 46
Airplane food, 155, 191
Airplanes, exercise on, 192
Airports, 192
Alcohol, 17, 34–35, 46, 156, 187, 189; and water, 187; calories in, 187; hangover cure, 188
Alertness, 121–22

Alfalfa, 114
Allergies, 151
Alley, Kirstie, 93
"Alligator skin," 243
Aloe powder, 114
Aloe vera, 115
Alzheimer's disease, 31
America Online, 220
American Dietetic Association, 4, 219
Amino acids, 111–12, 157, 239; uptake, 114
Androgen, 214
Animals, 52
Aniston, Jennifer, 87
Ankles, swollen, 120
Ann-Margret, 95
Antibiotics, alternative to, 122
Antioxidants, 47, 122, 237

Antiwrinkling, 62
Appetite suppressants, 114–19
Appetizers, 247
Apple cider vinegar, 82, 118
Apple crisp, 301
Apple nut cookies, 301
Apple shaped people, 76
Apples, 64, 170; red, 113
Applesauce, 60
Arby's, 59
Arugula and orange salad, 275
Aspartame, alternatives to, 118
Aspirin, 118
Auermann, Nadja, 84

B

Bagels, 60
Baked potato, 60
Baking, 47

Balance Bars, 214

Balance magazine, 216

Bananas, 27, 170

Barbie, 35

Bargains, 213–26

Bath towel, as ab machine, 131

Baywatch, 86

Bean soup, 268

Beans, 222

Beautiful Girls, 92

Bee pollen, 119

Beef eye of the round, 62

Beef tenderloin with onions, 284

Belts, 46, 68

Beta carotene, 121, 238

Beta-hydroxy-methylbutyrate (HMB), 111

Betting, 49

Beverages, carbonated, 104

Bicycle, stationary, 135

Bicycling, 254

Big clothes, 78

Binging, 9, 11, 154, 240

Biscotti, 302

Bissett, Josie, 91

Black bean and corn won ton cups, 261

Bladder wrack, 115

Bloating, 17, 73, 120, 151, 239, 251

Blood cholesterol, 237

Blood fat, 117

Blood flow, 73

Blood pressure, 52

Blood sugar, 150

Blueberries, 238

Blueberry cake, 304

Blueberry muffins, 296–97

Body fat, measuring, 4

Body lifts, 230

Body mass index, 5

Body shapers, 77

Body suit, 68

Body-Solid Exercise Equipment, 215

Boiling vegetables, 59

Books, as exercise equipment, 138

Boots, 77

Boredom, 7, 36, 145, 246

Bottles, as exercise equipment, 139

Bouillon, 48

Brain function, 57

Brandeis University, 111

Braxton, Toni, 92

Bread basket, 189

Bread, 26, 73, 150

Breakfast, 45, 54; skipping, 37, 147

Breast cancer, 237

Breast implants, 231

Breast lift, 232

Breast pockets, 76

Breast reduction, 231

Breath mints, 44

Breathing, 20, 44

Brinkley, Christie, 92

British Journal of Sports Medicine, 128

Bronzing powder, 70–72

Broomstick, as exercise equipment, 140

Brown sugar, 31

Budget, 160

Buffets, 184–86; plate size, 184

Burdock, 115

Burger King, 59

Butter, 31, 60, 245

Buttons, 68–69, 76

C

Cabbage diet, 98

Caffeine, 32, 233, 251

Cake, 60

Calcium, 61, 125, 251; supplements, 246

Calm atmosphere, 15

Calorie Control Council, 216

Calories, 22, 56; daily consumption, 253; insufficient, 37; limiting, 53; rationing, 57; underestimating, 4

Cancer, 31, 125

Candy, sugarless, 239

Candy wrappers, 46

Canned foods, refrigerating, 243

Capsicum, 115

Carbohydrate Addict's Official Home Page, 219

Carbohydrates, 28, 104

Carbonation, 104

Cardamom, 115

Career change, 50

Carrot bread, 297

Carrots and grapes, 278

Carrots, 238; glazed, 282

Carter, Lynda, 88

Cat's claw, 120

Cavities, preventing, 63

Cayenne, 116

Celebrities, secrets of, 81

Celery, 55, 61, 169, 247

Cellulite treatments, 232

Cereal, 26, 61, 63, 252, 256

Ch'i, 111, 115

Chairs, as exercise equipment, 137

Cheekbones, 70

Cheeks, 71

Cheese, 63, 253

Cheesecake cups, 303

Chewing, 242

Chicken, cholesterol in, 28

Chicken and pasta salad, 274–75

Chicken breast, 62

Chicken breasts, feta and mint, 287

Chicken salad, 269

Chickweed, 116

Children, 173–77; and eating disorders, 246; and weight, 173–77; genetic factors, 173; helping your child, 176–77; lifestyle, 174; self-image, 174; shared family behaviors, 175

Chili soup, 265

Chitosan, 109

Chocolate, 46; kisses, 303; truffles, 302

Choker, 68

Cholesterol, 28, 31, 121–22, 161

Christmas, 181

Chromium picolinate, 109, 112

Cinnamon, 116, 170

Circulation, 115–17, 124

Citrus salad, 270

Cleavage, faking, 72

Clothes, buying small, 79

Clothing: expressing personality, 79; too tight, 168

Coenzyme Q10, 110

Coffee, 32, 45, 61, 63, 157, 169, 248; calories in, 241; flavored, 48

Cole slaw, 272

Collagen, 238

Collins, Joan, 103

Colon cancer, 131

Colon cleanse, 82

Colonic irrigation, 152

Color: effect on appetite, 36, 45; of food, 47

Comfort foods, 7, 9–10, 26

Competition, 51

Compliments, 41

Concealer, 72

Conjugated linoleic acid (CLA), 110

Constipation, 157

Contract, 10

Cookies, 20; low fat, 21

Cooking: for the family, 159–60; on a budget, 222–23; temperature, 48

Corsets, 34

Cosmetic surgery, 227

Cottage cheese, 63

Cotton, 68

Couscous salad, 272

Cox, Courtney, 89, 158

Crab meat spread, 263

Cramps, 120

Crash diets, 97

Cravings, 7, 30, 46, 49, 54, 63, 89, 145, 249; eliminating, 148–50

Crawford, Cindy, 83

Cream cheese, 60

Cream, 60

Creatine, 110, 214

Creativity, effect of exercise on, 128

Crisco, 156

Crisp bread, 299

Cross trainer, 136

Cucumber salad with dill, 275–76

Cuffs, 68

Curtis, Jamie Lee, 92

Custard, 305

Cyber Diet, 216

Cyber Kitchen, 216

Cystein, 239

D

Daily caloric intake, 4

Daily journal, 4, 162

Daily schedule, 18

Dairy products, 83

Dairy Queen, 58

Dancing, 133–34

Dandelion root, 116
Dandelion tea, 82
Dang gui, 120
Dateline, 86
Days of Our Lives, 90
Decorations, edible, 182
Deja News, 222
Deli salad, 273
Deprivation, 3, 9
Dessert, 17, 63
DHEA, 214
Diabetes, 237, 252
Diaz, Cameron, 93
Diet books, 6
Diet City, 217
Diet clubs, 22, 225
Diet programs, 6; complex, 6
Diet scale, 43
Diet shot, 35
Diet soup, 98
Diet supplements, 21

Dieting: and motherhood, 193; fear of, 2; myths, 21–38; reasons for, 19
Dieting gimmicks, 255
Diets: failure of, 1–2; high protein, 29; overdoing, 35; starting, 2
Digestion, 115–17
Dill, 170
Dining out, 188–90
Discount Natural Foods, 214
Diuretic, 82, 114–17, 251
DNA, 120
Dog, 52
Double chin, 70–71
Doughnuts, 306
Dr. Atkins' Diet Revolution, 100
Drescher, Fran, 70, 87
Dressing, rules of, 67
Driver, Minnie, 86
Driving, 150, 191
Dunaway, Faye, 96
Dynasty, 96

E

Ear, pinching, 41
Earrings, 30, 68
Easter, 188
Eating: and exercise, 247; constant, 246; enjoyment of, 9; frequency, 40; late night, 241; regularly, 25; sitting down, 15; standing up, 29; triggers, 48; with music, 36
Eating by the clock, 4
Ebony, 94
Echinacea, 120
Eden, Barbara, 96
Egg drop soup, 265
Eggplant, tomatoes, and feta, 291–92
Eggs, 31, 62, 170, 239
Elle, 10
Emergency measures, 104
Emotional eating, 94
Emotional pain, 26
Empire styles, 76

Enchiladas, 293

Endermologie, 233

Energy bars, 37

Energy, 25, 39, 116, 120, 125

Envy, 51

Epaulets, 76

Ephedra (ma huang), 116

Evangelista, Linda, 84

Evans, Linda, 96

Evening primrose oil, 120

Exercise equipment, 127, 134; alternatives to, 136–40; buying, 215; renting, 225

Exercise videos, 140

Exercise, 4, 127–141, 152; and motherhood, 193; form, 33; on a budget, 223–225; quality of, 134; special clothing, 31; time of, 128, 247; with partner, 168

Exfoliator, 72

Expectations, 20

Eyebrows, 71

Eyes, emphasizing, 71

Eyesight, 124

F

Fabrics, choosing, 68

Face, drawing attention to, 68

Face powder, translucent, 71

Failure, 13

False hunger, 148

Family dynamics, 175

Family roots, 50

Family, 50, 144

Fast food, 58, 153; serving size, 58

Fasting, 22, 32

Fat test, 240

"Fat thinking", 148

Fat, 46; calorie content, 62; limiting, 104; weight of, 252

Fatigue, 7

Fen-phen, 112

Fennel, 116

Feta and mint chicken breasts, 287

Fiber, 45, 61, 109, 151, 157, 183, 254; tablets, 33

Figs, 170

Fillers, low calorie, 66

Fish, 185; cholesterol in, 28

Fisher, Joely, 85

Fitness Discount Outlet, 215

Fitness Online, 217

Fitness Partner Connection, 217

Flank steak, 284–85

Flax seed, 116

Fleming, Peggy, 94

Flossing, 53

Fluid retention, 73

Folic acid, 120

Food: as a love affair, 54; as antidote, 9; choices, 53, 57–66; cold, 242; container size, 42; daily choices, 64; grating, 243; high calorie, 66; labeling, 248; packaging, 46; portioning, 238; quality of, 53

Frederique, 91

Free radicals, 121, 125, 237
Freeda Vitamins, Inc., 214
Friends, 47, 50, 52, 87, 89, 129, 144
Frozen fruit pops, 63
Frozen yogurt, 21
Fruit, with hard skin, 243
Fruit juices, 254
Fruit skewers with mango purée, 306
Fruits, 57; fat-free, 104
Fuentes, Daisy, 84

G

Gabor, Ava, 6
Garcinia cambogia, 111, 116
Gardening, 128, 132, 224
Garlic and papaya diet, 235–36
Garlic, 121
Gastric surgery, 228–30
Gazpacho, 266
German potato salad, 271
Gibbons, Leeza, 87
Gifts, 182

Ginger snaps, 86
Ginger, 121
Ginkgo biloba, 121
Ginsana, 215
Ginseng, 122, 170
Giving in, 48
Glands, 26
Glucuronic acid, 122
Glutamine, 111, 113
Goals, 3, 11, 21, 23–24, 130
Good Health Web, 217
Good Morning America, 87
Grains, 57
Granola, 61
Grape seeds, 122
Grape-Nuts, 61
Grapefruit diet, 99
Grapefruit seed extract, 122
Grapes, 47
Greek salad, 269
Green tea, 116, 171
Griffith, Melanie, 88, 103

Guarana, 117
Gum, 73
Gymnema tea, 117

H

Habits, 24
Hair: lightening, 70; restoration, 120
Hair styling, 69; blow drying, 70; for double chins, 70; for round faces, 69; height of, 70; highlights, 70; layers, 69; upswept hairdo, 70
Hall, Deidre, 90
Ham and cheddar bites, 264
Handbag, 75, 77
Hands, elongating, 71
Hangover cure, 188
Hash browns, 279
Hawn, Goldie, 96
Hawthorn, 117
Hayek, Salma, 92
Headaches, 8, 123
Health clubs, 193

Healthy Choice Kitchen, 217
Healthy Ideas, 217
Heart disease, 122, 237
Heart Information Network, 219
Heels, 72, 77
Henner, Marilu, 93
Hepburn, Audrey, 85
Herbs, 41, 114
High blood pressure, 121
High protein diet, 100
HMB, 111
Hobby, 50
Hoffman-LaRoche, 111
Holidays, 12, 179–94
Home Arts, 218
Homeopathic healing, 125
Honey, 171
Hotel, exercise at, 192
Housework, 95, 128, 224
Hunger, 148
Hutton, Lauren, 84
Hydration, 39

Hydroxyl citric acid, 111
Hygiene, 167
Hypertension, 133

I

I Dream of Jeannie, 96
Ice water, 82, 236
Ideal weight, 2
Immune system, 120, 122–23
Injury, 140
Insulin, 32, 73
Intelihealth, 220
International Breath Institute, 44
Internet Resources, 215–22
Internet Support Groups, 220–21
Intimacy, 165–72
Iron, 122
Italian dressing, 277

J

Jacket, 68; long, 68
Jackson, Janet, 94

Jell-O, 44, 63, 254
Jelly beans, 83
Jelly, 60
Jet lag, 123
Johns Hopkins University, 19, 54, 220
Johnsen, Kristen, 93
Judd, Ashley, 86
Juice Fast, 97
Jump rope, 45, 132, 191
Junk food, 25, 159

K

Kansas State University, 128
Karan, Donna, 103
Kava, 117
Kellogg's Corn Pops, 254
Kelp, 82, 117
Kentucky Fried Chicken, 58
Kitchen step-stool, 131
Kitt, Eartha, 96, 130
Knits, 69

Knots Landing, 95
Kola nut, 117
Kombucha mushroom, 122
Koop, C. Everett, 216
Kramer, Kathy, 225
Kudrow, Lisa, 91
Kyolic, 215

L

L-carnitine, 112
Labels, food content, 41
Lamb shank, 62
Late night munchies, 156
Laughing, 41
Lavender oil, 123
Lavender, 171
Lawrence, Sharon, 92
Laxatives, 114–18, 152
Leek dip, 262
Legginess, 77
Lemon bars, 300
Lemon chicken, 286

Lemon pepper popovers, 296
Lemons, 171
Lettuce, 47, 66; color of, 63
Licorice root, 123
LifeSavers, 83
Light mayonnaise, 255
Lighting, flattering, 170
Lights, intensity of, 54
Lingerie, 77
Lipase, 112
Lipids, 121
Liposuction, 227–28
Lipstick, 246
Liquid diet, 100
Little City, 86
Lobster shells, 109
Lollipops, 240
Loofah, 238
Loren, Sophia, 94
Louis-Dreyfus, Julia, 90
Low fat foods, 29, 57, 144
Low Fat Lifestyle Forum, 218

Lucci, Susan, 90
Lunden, Joan, 87
Lycra, 68

M

Macpherson, Elle, 84
Macrobiotic diet, 94
Magnesium, 61; deficiency, 7
Magnetic wellness products, 30
Mail order catalogs, 52
Makeup tips, 71
Male breast reduction, 232
Mansfield, Jayne, 85
Manz, Esther, 226
Margarine, 31, 245
Marriage, and weight, 246
Marshmallow creme, 60
Mascara, 71
Mashed potatoes, 180
Mayo Clinic, 218
Mayonnaise, 60
McDonald's, 59

McDowell, Andie, 94
McGraw, Ali, 96
Meals: regular, 152; skipping, 14, 241
Measurements, recording, 43
Meat loaf, 285–86
Meats, 223, 248; cut, 62
Meditation, 242
Melatonin, 123
Melrose Place, 91
Memory, 121
Men's Fitness Online, 218
Menopause, 120
Menstrual cycles, 7, 28, 34, 157, 252
Meridia, 112
MET-Rx, 214–15
Metabolism, 39–40, 54, 82, 105, 115–17, 124, 250
Microwaves, 32
Microwaving vegetables, 59
Milk: in coffee, 63; skim, 60, 248
Milk cartons, as exercise equipment, 131

Miller, Penelope Ann, 86
Mini meal diet, 101
Minimizers, 74
Mirror, 51, 238
Model's diet, 98
Models, secrets of, 81
Moisturizing cream, 72
Molasses cookies, 307
Money, 22
Monochromatic dressing, 68
Monroe, Marilyn, 85
Moore, Demi, 86
Motion sickness, 121
Motivation, 22, 250
Movies, snacking at, 254
Muffins, 30, 296
Muscle, weight of, 252
Mushrooms, 171, 239, 259
Music, 36
Mussels, 171
Mustard, 60

N
Nail polish, 71
Nap, 26
Natural diet pills, 249
Nausea, 121
Necklines, 68
Negative calories, 82, 247
Nestle Sweet Success, 100
Net Loss Club, 225
New England Journal of Medicine, 153
Newsgroups, health and fitness, 221
Nolin, Gena Lee, 86
Nonfat foods, 32
Noodle salad, 271
Nouvelle cuisine, 49
Nutmeg, 171
Nutrition Analysis Tool, 218
NYPD Blue, 92

O
Oatmeal, 222

Olive oil, 251
Onion rings, 263
Onion tart, 298
Onion twists, 299
Orange liqueur, 64
Orange marmalade, 64
Orange-glazed asparagus, 281
Orlistat, 112
Osmond, Marie, 85
Overeaters Anonymous, 55, 225–26
Overeating, triggers, 4
Oysters rockefeller, 289
Oysters, 171

P

Pace, 3
Packaged foods, 34
Palazzo styling, 77
Panties, tummy toning, 78
Pants, slim, 77
Pantyhose, 68, 77; slimming, 78
Papaya, 117, 235

Parsley, 117, 171
Parties, 182
Parton, Dolly, 87; diet, 98
Party mix, 186
Passion foods, 170–72
Pasta diet, 107
Pasta primavera, 295
Pasta, 59, 73, 222
Pauley, Jane, 86
Pea Salad, 270
Peaches, 171
Peanut oil, 251
Pear shaped people, 76
Peas and onions, 280
Pendant, 76
Peppers, vegetarian stuffed, 294
Perfume, 46
Personality, 79
Phen cal, 106, 112
Phenylalanine, 113, 118
Phillips, Michelle, 95
Phosphorus, 125

Phyllium, 117
Physicians, 1, 128
Pill, 246
Pimples, 63
Pineapple steak kabobs, 285
Pita chips, 63
Pizza bread, 297–98
Pizza potato skins, 259–60
Pizza, 64, 255
Plate color, 45
Plateaus, 53, 161–63, 249
Playboy, 90
PMS, 120
Pockets, 68–69
Polysaccharides, 120
Popcorn mix, southwestern, 261
Popcorn, 44, 64
Popovers, 296
Pork chop, 62
Pork steaks with peppercorn glaze, 286
Pork tenderloin, 62

Portion, size of, 65

Portions, 183, 238; measuring, 43, 56; size, 241

Portobello-stuffed zucchini boats, 260

Posture, 53, 69

Potassium, 27

Potato salad, 271

Potatoes, 256

Power, 3

Pregnenolone, 113

Prescription weight loss supplements, 21

Pretzels, 63; fat-free, 21

Prevention, 217

Prints: floral, 68; on clothing, 68

Protein Power, 100

Protein, 27, 62, 93, 104, 150, 242; sources of, 73, 253

Pudding, 63

Pycnogenol, 123

Pyruvate, 113

Q

QVC Shopping Network, 85

R

Raisin Bran, 61

Ranch dressing, 277

Raspberries, 171

Rayon, 68

Reaction time, 57

Redux, 112

Reflexology, 248

Refrigerator, 39, 162, 238

Resolutions, 10

Respiratory problems, 120

Rest, 150

Reward system, 8

Riboflavin, 62

Rice almondine, 282

Rice cakes, 44, 55

Rice, 66

Rinna, Lisa, 94

RNA, 120

Roberts, Julia, 88

Romance, 134

Rosemary "Fries", 280

Ross, Diana, 95, 130

Rowing machine, 136

Royal jelly, 123

Rules, breaking, 20

Running, 133, 224

Russell, Jane, 85

S

S'mores fudge, 305

Saccharin, alternatives to, 118

Safflower oil, 251

Salmon, 239

Salsa dip, 259

Salsa, 44, 60

Salt, 73, 249

Sarong skirt, 69

Saunas, 32

Scallops, 171; baked, 289

Scarsdale Diet, 100

Scarves, as exercise equipment, 138
Scents, 166
Schiffer, Claudia, 84
School lunches, 176
Science of Obesity and Weight Control, 220
Seafood bisque, 290
Seasonal challenges, 12
Seasonal-affective disorder, 153
Seaweed, 124
Seed-containing fruits, 237
Seinfield, 90
Selenium, 62, 124, 156, 239
Self-acceptance, 169
Self-esteem, 23, 37
Self-perception, 165
Self-permission, 6
Self-tanner, 73
Selfishness, 47
Senna, 118
Serving size, 56
Sesame broccoli and cauliflower, 281

Setbacks, 23, 158
Sex, 165; and headaches, 166; and menstruation, 166; and mental ability, 166; and skin tone, 166; as exercise, 166; effect on cholesterol, 166
Seymour, Jane, 87
Shape magazine, 218
Shirts: cut of, 67; oversized, 76
Shoes: low heeled, 68; sturdy, 69
Shopping, 242
Shorts, 76
Shoulder pads, 69
Shredded Wheat, 61
Shrimp, deviled, 290
Sibutramine, 113
Simmons, Richard, 219
Skim milk custard, 305
Skin hydration, 124
Skin, 124–25; sagging, 156
Skirt: A-line, 67; dirndl, 77; front-slit, 77; length of, 69; pencil, 77

Sleeping pill, 123
Sleeping, 242
Slimfast, 100
Slips, 78
Smell, sense of, 45
Smith, Anna Nicole, 90
Smith, Jaclyn, 88
Smoking, 154
Snacking, 152; budget, 44
Snacks, low calorie, 58
Snow peas and carrots, 278
Soap stars, secrets of, 90
Social situations, 17
Socks, 77
Soda bottles, as exercise equipment, 131
Soda, 32, 73; diet, 251
Sodium, 73, 104
Somers, Suzanne, 87
Soreness, 250
Sorvino, Mira, 92
Soup cans, as exercise equipment, 131

Soup, 60, 223

Soy, 237

Spa 3-day diet, 105

Spices, 60, 152

Spicy foods, 236

Spider veins, 122

Spinach artichoke dip, 258

Spinach dip, 262

Spinach salad, 273

Spirituality, 55, 86

Spirulina, 118

Sports, family, 193

Sports drinks, 21

Sports Illustrated, 14

Spot exercising, 31, 250

Sprouts, 66

St. John's Wort, 119, 214

Stair stepper, 45, 49, 127, 135–36

Stamina, 249

Starches, 73

Stationary bicycle, 49

Steaming vegetables, 59

Stevia, 118

Stewardess diet, 98

Stomach, shrinking, 240

Straw, 73

Streamlining activities, 56

Strength gyms, 136

Stress, 7, 12, 41, 52, 117, 123, 146

Striptease, 86

Stuffing, 180

Subliminal tapes, 30

Substitutions, 60

Subway, 58

Sugar addictions, 154

Sugar and spice doughnuts, 306

Sugar, 31, 60, 251; powdered, 60

Sun damage, 123

Sun-related diseases, 125

Sunflower oil, 251

Sunflower seeds, 172

Supermarket carts, 42

Supplements, 21, 109–25; buying, 214–15

Support, 18

Surgeries, weight-related, 231–32

Swallowing, 46

Sweet potatoes, 62

Sweet tooth, 54, 117

Swim wear, 74; color of, 75; patterns, 75; sizes, 74

Swiss asparagus au gratin, 283

T

Tailoring, 78

Take Off Pounds Sensibly (TOPS), 226

Taste buds, 41; inhibitor, 33

Taylor, Niki, 83

Tea, 32, 48

Teeth, brushing, 43, 53, 133, 149, 184

Temptation, 49

Thanksgiving, 179–81

Therapy, 26

Thermogenesis, 115–16, 118, 237

Thyroid function, 115, 117

Tiegs, Cheryl, 89
Titanic, 93
Toast, 249
Tofu with vegetables, stir-fried, 291
Tomato soup, 60
Tomato, 66
Tonalin, 110
Tootsie Pop, 61
Tortellini soup, 267
Tortillas, 292
Toxins, 32, 44
Travel, 190; exercise during, 191
Treadmill, 45, 49, 128, 135
Trousers, pleated, 67
True Lies, 92
Tryptophan, 113
Tummy tuck, 231
Tuna with tomato vinaigrette, 288
Turkey meat loaf, 288
Turkey spirals, mediterranean, 287
Turkey, 180
Turner, Tina, 95

Twin Lab, 215
Tyrosine, 113

U

Ulcers, 121, 123
Universal, 215
University of Wisconsin-Madison, 23
Uplift shapers, 78
USA Today, 219
USDA, 4

V

Vacation brochures, 52
Vacations, 158, 179–94
Valentine's Day, 188
Valerian root, 118
Vanadyl sulfate, 114
Vegetable cans, as exercise equipment, 138
Vegetable salad, 276
Vegetable soup, 268
Vegetable tortillas, 292

Vegetables, 57; fat-free, 104; grilled, 30; with hard skin, 243
Vest, 68
Vichyssoise, 267
Victoria's Secret, 91
Videos, exercise, 224
Vinaigrette, 60
Vinegar, 118
Visualization, 15
Vitamin A, 62, 121, 124, 239
Vitamin absorption, 123
Vitamin B complex, 239
Vitamin B-1 (Thiamine), 124
Vitamin B, 124
Vitamin C, 123, 125
Vitamin Connection, 214
Vitamin D, 125
Vitamin E, 123–25, 156
Vitamin House, 215
Vitamin K, 62
Vitamin Shoppe, 215

Vitamins, 28, 32, 119–25; buying, 214–15; natural, 29

W

Waldorf salad, 274
Walking, 39, 130–31, 224
Wall, as exercise equipment, 139
Warm liquids, 48
Water retention, 249
Water weight reduction, 114
Water, 39, 82, 105, 151, 157, 251
Weider, 215
Weight, ideal, 5–6, 11
Weight gain, false, 43
Weight loss industry, 13
Weight problems, glandular, 26
Welch, Raquel, 95
Wendy's, 59
Wheat germ, 63
Wheat grass juice, 125
Williams, Vanessa, 87
Willpower, 47, 143

Wine vinegar, 60
Wine, 172, 254; red, 240
Winslet, Kate, 93
Winter, 12, 153
Woolens, 68

Y

Yahoo, 222
Yams, 239
Yellow pepper and orange soup, 266
Yo yo dieting, 16
Yogurt, 60, 63, 239
Yukon Strength Training Equipment, 215

Z

Zone, The, 100
Zucchini boats, 260
Zucchini frittata, 279–80